HYSTERECTOMY

Hysterectomy

A COMPLETE, UP-TO-DATE GUIDE
TO EVERYTHING ABOUT IT AND WHY
IT MAY BE NEEDED

Nancy Nugent

INTRODUCTION BY MYRON I. BUCHMAN, M.D.

DRAWINGS BY WALTER R. NUGENT

DOUBLEDAY & COMPANY, INC., GARDEN CITY, NEW YORK
1976

LIBRARY OF CONGRESS CATALOGING IN PUBLICATION DATA
NUGENT, NANCY.
HYSTERECTOMY: A COMPLETE, UP-TO-DATE GUIDE TO EVERYTHING
ABOUT IT AND WHY IT MAY BE NEEDED.
INCLUDES INDEX.
1. HYSTERECTOMY.   I. TITLE.   [DNLM: 1. HYSTERECTOMY—
POPULAR WORKS. WP468 N967H]
RG391.N83   618.1′453
ISBN: 0-385-03887-9
LIBRARY OF CONGRESS CATALOG CARD NUMBER 75–36605

Contents

Introduction

A pregnant woman today has many books, periodicals, and manuals available to her explaining her physical and emotional development during the course of her gestation. However, when a woman faces the prospect of an operative procedure such as a hysterectomy, there is little or nothing to which she can refer except complex medical texts written in technical language understood only by trained professionals.

This book fills the gap. For such a woman, it covers carefully, precisely, and simply the reasons for a hysterectomy, and explains the type of operative procedure that is carried out.

Hysterectomy outlines the manner in which a woman is prepared in the hospital, the operating room regimen, and the postoperative treatment. It contains personal experiences of actual women the author has interviewed, and it is flavored with case histories showing attitudes and feelings that patients harbored before and after the operative procedure.

It will stimulate thought, allay fears, and dispel superstitions that may plague the prospective candidate for a hysterectomy.

Although the medical aspects of the book have been carefully researched and written, there are undoubtedly variations in procedures from hospital to hospital, and the choice and indications for the operation are tailored to the individual patient.

This book will be of great help to the patient who faces the prospect of a hysterectomy—and to the physician, who also realizes that the subject is so varied and so enormous that he could not possibly anticipate all the questions the patient may have before she enters the hospital and during the course of her illness and recovery.

Myron I. Buchman, M.D.
New York, N. Y.

HYSTERECTOMY

CHAPTER 1

What Is Hysterectomy?

As USUAL, the Greeks had the words for it:

hystera   ektome

The suffix "ectomy" is applied to all words that name surgical operations in which organs are removed from the body. The word is derived from the Greek *ektome*, meaning "excision."

Ektome, in turn, is a combination of *ex*, meaning "out of," and *tome*, meaning "a cutting." Thus, when the appendix is taken out the patient undergoes an appendectomy, removal of the tonsils is a tonsillectomy, and so on.

Hystera is the Greek word for uterus, or womb. Interestingly, it is also the source of the word "hysteria," meaning ranting, raving, and outlandish behavior in general. Many ancient civilizations believed that, since new human life came out of the womb, the organ must be bewitched. Because of their wombs, women were for centuries both revered for their life-giving qualities and put down for being "different."

"Different" from what? From men, of course, and since men did not have wombs, they were considered "normal."

Why? Because they, the men, were doing all the considering in those days and were not yet ready to accept the concept of differences within the realm of normality. Sauce for the gander was all the sauce you got—for a very long time.

Men, too, did not go through what they believed was the "curious and unnatural" process of bleeding once a month—for which women were considered unclean. In some civilizations, a menstruating woman was thought to be a temporary sorceress, to be feared and banished to isolation until her period was over.

The uterus was also thought (at least by the early, word-coining Greeks) to be the very center of a woman's being and the sole source of her personality. Thus, any female behavior that incurred the disapproval of men was attributed to the eerie influences of the demons residing in the uterus and was termed "hysterical." Interesting that the term has survived—even though what we now call hysterical behavior has its basis in psychology rather than reproductive anatomy, we continue to use terminology that directly links it to the womb. Technically, there should be no such thing as an hysterical man, but such are the vagaries of language.

Putting this all together, we come up with *hysterectomy*, literally the surgical removal of the uterus.

The extent to which this operation is performed depends on many factors, primarily the extent of the disease that has damaged and/or destroyed the uterus and must be removed. A partial hysterectomy, obviously, is excision of only a portion of the womb. A total hysterectomy concerns the entire uterus, and portions of the Fallopian tubes and ovaries may or may not be removed at the same time, depending again on the nature and extent of the disease.

The physical results of hysterectomy vary according to

what and how much is taken out. The emotional results seem limitless and dependent on each woman's circumstances and psyche. But the undeniable fact that the patient will never again be able to give birth to a child places on hysterectomy an onus not shared by other forms of surgery. It is frequently viewed with dread and alarm, and both patient and physician may find themselves faced with emotional problems often as serious as physical considerations.

The entire internal set of female reproductive organs has been regarded through history as the very center of life itself. It has been mercilessly abused by both neglect and maltreatment, and, at the same time, worshiped and revered. Small wonder that surgical mutilation of this system, even when performed as a life-saving measure, has been the source of severe emotional trauma for so many women.

Much soul-searching and counseling surround the anticipation, performance, and aftermath of the hysterectomy, and the decision to go through with it is seldom, if ever, taken lightly, even by those few women who request the operation for birth-control reasons.

The belief that a thorough understanding of the physical and emotional aspects of hysterectomy can be both helpful and reassuring to the patient, her family, and her friends is the basis of this work.

CHAPTER 2

The Basic Anatomy

A GOOD WORKING KNOWLEDGE of the female reproductive system is a prerequisite to understanding the hysterectomy. Most women are pretty well informed about what's going on in this area; nonetheless, a review of the basic facts should be helpful.

There are two sets of female reproductive organs, the internal set and the external; we are concerned with the internal set, which consists of the ovaries, the Fallopian tubes, the uterus, the cervix, and the vagina.

THE OVARIES

The two ovaries, located in the lower abdomen—one to the right and one to the left of the uterus—produce the human egg (ovum) and the female hormones estrogen and progesterone. The ovaries are rounded in shape, much like a medicinal capsule, and are approximately an inch and a half long and about three quarters of an inch wide. They are not, as is often thought, directly connected to the uterus by the Fallopian tubes. Rather they are held in place by ligaments and are contiguous with, or in close proximity to, the tubes (*see Figures 1 and 2*). The *fimbria,* or fringelike ends of the tubes, envelop the ovaries, which lie beneath and behind the arches of their Fallopian tubes. Their position is not exact, however, since they are often displaced by the expansion of the uterus during pregnancy.

Inside each ovary are numerous ball-shaped follicles, each containing a single ovum. These follicles secrete the hormones, estrogen and progesterone, that prepare the body for pregnancy and prevent the ovaries from releasing additional eggs during the nine months of gestation. During the reproductive years, the supply of follicles is constantly maintained by the body—the ovaries do not "run out" of them, even though one is "used up" each month.

At the beginning of each menstrual cycle, or approximately every twenty-eight days (except during pregnancy or when ovulation is inhibited by oral contraceptives), one follicle begins to mature. It becomes enlarged, and the ovum within it becomes surrounded by fluid and by a protective capsule that is attached to the wall of the follicle.

As it matures, the follicle moves within the ovary until it is situated at the periphery, at which point it begins to protrude through the ovarian wall. While the follicle is moving, the ovum within it gradually detaches itself from the follicle's wall.

When the follicle has reached the proper position, its wall ruptures, and the ovum is catapulted out of the ovary. (Often, women have claimed that they can *feel* the follicle burst, and this is called *mittelschmerz,* or ovulation pain.) What was once the follicle then becomes known as the *corpus luteum.*

The continuing role of the corpus luteum depends upon whether or not the released ovum becomes fertilized. If it does not, and is absorbed and passed out of the body with the menstrual fluid, the corpus luteum has no further function; it merges with the inner surface of the ovary and disappears.

When pregnancy occurs, however, the corpus luteum is needed to provide the preparatory functions that will later be taken over by the placenta (afterbirth)—the nourishment and maintenance of the fetus. Just after the follicle bursts, the point of rupture seals itself, and the corpus luteum becomes filled with proliferating cells and blood. It grows to about three times its original size and functions until about the fourth month of pregnancy. During that time it manufactures and releases hormones for three specific purposes. First, these hormones regulate the implantation of the fertilized egg in the lining of the uterus and determine its healthy growth. Second, they stimulate the mammary glands (breasts) to enlarge and produce milk. And third, the hormones inhibit the normal function of the ovaries so that no more eggs will be released until after the birth. When the baby is breast-fed, this inhibition usually continues until the child has been weaned, though it is not a foolproof method of birth control.

After the placenta has assumed these functions, the corpus luteum regresses slowly, sometimes lasting until the termination of pregnancy. Eventually it disappears into the ovarian wall, as it would have if pregnancy had not occurred.

THE FALLOPIAN TUBES

When the ovum has been expelled from the ovary, it passes through the ovarian fimbria and into the large, hornlike opening of the Fallopian tube.

The two tubes, one on each side of the uterus, extend outward from the top of the uterus and curve over the ovaries like protective tree branches (*see Figures 1 and 2*). Each

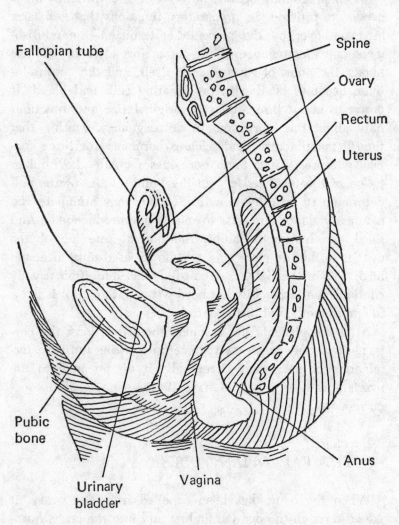

Figure 1

tube curves downward at the end, and the tissue spreads out like the end of a horn. The sole purpose of the Fallopian tube is to provide the egg with a pathway to the uterus and, it is believed, a hospitable place for fertilization. If the ovum is destined to unite with a sperm cell, this will probably take place within the Fallopian tube, after which the fertilized ovum will proceed through the tube to the uterus and become implanted in the uterine wall. Occasionally, though rarely, the ovum becomes embedded in the tube at the point of fertilization: this is called *ectopic* or tubal pregnancy and requires surgical intervention since the narrow tube cannot accommodate the growing embryo for very long.

THE UTERUS

The uterus is a somewhat inverted pear-shaped organ located in the middle of the lower abdomen, behind the urinary bladder and in front of the rectum. In its nonpregnant state, it is about three inches long; during pregnancy, it expands like a balloon to accommodate the growth of the fetus or fetuses it holds. Its top opens on either side to the Fallopian tubes, and its bottom opens through the uterine cervix into the vagina. Its walls are thick and muscular and are lined with a mucous membrane called the *endometrium*. Viewed from the side, in its nonpregnant state, the uterus normally tips forward, generally over the bladder (*Figure 1*). When pregnant, it exhibits extraordinary stretching ability, expanding to approximately sixteen or more times its nonpregnant size—and even more in cases of multiple birth.

In its nonpregnant state, the inside of the uterus is a triangular-shaped hollow, spreading out to the two Fallopian tubes at the top, and narrowing to the cervix at the bottom. The muscular substance of the uterine wall, called the myometrium, is the supporting structure of the uterus. During the menstrual cycle, a thick, rich coating builds up on the endometrium, which lines the inside surface of the myometrium. If the ovum is fertilized, it will embed itself in this coating when it reaches the uterus and be nourished by it throughout pregnancy. If the ovum is not fertilized by the time it reaches the uterus, the coating will disintegrate and pass out of the body as menstrual fluid, carrying the ovum with it. As soon as menstruation begins, a new coating starts to form on the endometrium in preparation for the next month's ovum.

THE CERVIX

The Latin word *cervix* means "neck"; thus, the uterine cervix is literally the neck of the uterus, the part that extends into the vagina. The vaginal part (*Figure 2*), which surrounds the actual opening of the uterus into the vagina, includes a thick, soft "collar" of tissue that is often thought to be the cervix in its entirety, but is not.

The cervix admits the sperm-carrying seminal fluid into the uterus for possible fertilization and, when a baby is about to be born, becomes the beginning of the birth canal. At that time it opens, or dilates, slowly, centimeter by centimeter, until the opening is wide enough for the uterine contractions to push the baby through on its way to the outside world. Once the baby has been born, it opens again to eject the placenta, then returns (over a period of days) to its original size. During the monthly menstrual period, the menstrual fluid takes the same route, passing through the cervix and vagina and out of the body.

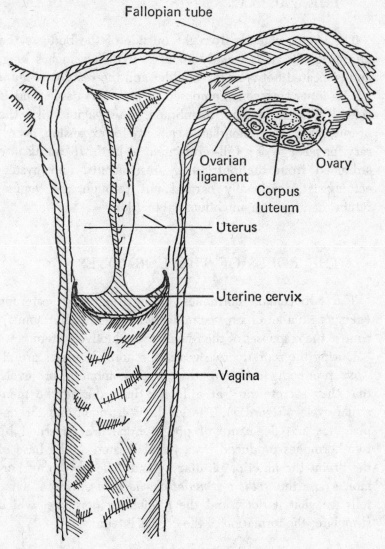

Figure 2

THE VAGINA

The vagina extends from the outside of the body to the uterine cervix; it is usually about four to five inches long, and is located between the bladder and the rectum (*Figure 1*). Its inner surface is composed of muscular tissue, and is coated with a mucous membrane. The vagina, like the uterus, possesses a remarkable capacity for expansion, necessary for passage of a full-term infant at birth. It can also be stretched from the outside by instruments, and hysterectomy is occasionally carried out through the vagina, rather than through an abdominal incision.

THE ROLES OF THE HORMONES

The two female hormones, estrogen and progesterone (along with a lot of very complicated subsidiary hormones), control the responses of the female reproductive system.

During the reproductive years, the normal ovaries are always producing estrogen, though the amounts, or levels, that they secrete vary at different times during the menstrual cycle (*Figure 3*). The levels of estrogen and the appearance and departure of progesterone are governed by two hormones produced by a gland located at the base of the brain—the anterior pituitary gland. The governing hormones are the *follicle-stimulating hormone*, whose name tells us what it does, and the *luteinizing hormone*, which stimulates the formation of the corpus luteum.

As menstrual bleeding begins the follicle-stimulating hormone signals the ovaries to produce a moderate amount of estrogen, which will cause the endometrium to proliferate, or become enlarged (progesterone is not present at this time). The estrogen level continues to increase for a few days, as the endometrium builds up in preparation for receiving a fertilized egg. As the ovum begins to push its way out of the follicle, the levels of estrogen and luteinizing hormone increase sharply and steadily, reaching a peak just before the follicle is ruptured and the egg expelled.

As the estrogen level reaches its peak the follicle, which will soon become the corpus luteum, begins to secrete a small amount of progesterone (*Figure 3*). This is the hormone that plays a major part in preparing the body for pregnancy. Its level increases steadily over the next few days as the follicle ruptures and the ovum makes its way into the Fallopian tube in anticipation of fertilization.

If the ovum is not fertilized, the corpus luteum begins its regression and releases less and less progesterone each day. The estrogen level decreases at the same time until, as bleeding begins, the amount of estrogen being secreted is again moderate. By this time, the progesterone level has tapered off to practically nothing, and soon there will be none at all.

Figure 3 shows the comparative levels of the hormones at different stages during the cycle, and the growth and recession of the endometrium when pregnancy does not occur.

When pregnancy occurs, the levels of estrogen and progesterone remain high throughout the nine months of gestation, both dropping off sharply at the time of birth.

When the roles of the hormones in the menstrual cycle

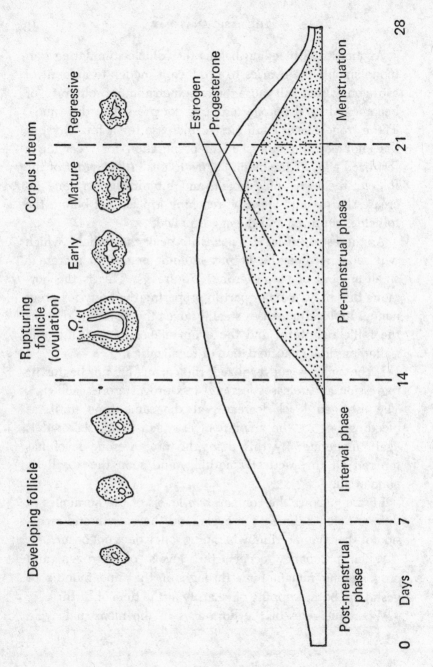

Figure 3

are understood, it can easily be seen that abnormalities and imbalances in their levels can cause mild to serious consequences—some of which will be described in the following chapters.

CHAPTER 3

Why Hysterectomy Is Performed: Fibroid Tumors and Endometriosis

---

HYSTERECTOMY IS USUALLY performed as a last-ditch measure, particularly when the patient is young and it may be possible to preserve her ability to bear children by resorting to other types of treatment or alternate surgical procedures. There are instances in which a patient will request the operation as the ultimate measure in birth control, or to be rid of potentially precancerous tissue along with existing non-malignant tumors. Most hysterectomies, however, are performed only after the gynecologist has rejected every other possible form of correcting a potentially dangerous condition.

FIBROID TUMORS—WHAT ARE THEY?

Although popular opinion holds that the majority of hysterectomies are performed to remove cancer, it is actually the fibroid tumor that is responsible in most cases—and a fibroid tumor usually is not cancer. It is, however, the most common tumor found in women.

The word "tumor" is defined by Dorland's Medical Dictionary as "a mass of new tissue that persists and grows independently of its surrounding structures, and has no physiologic use." The dictionary then goes on for three columns with definitions of different kinds of tumors, among them the fibroid: "a tumor composed of fibrous or fully developed connective tissue." This means simply that the fibroid tumor is a useless lump made up of fibers, or elongated structures of tissue.

Fibroid tumors can grow almost anywhere in the body, including on the skin, but we are concerned here solely with those that originate in the folds of the inner surface of the uterus—known as uterine fibroids. They can be small or can grow so large that the shape of the uterus—and sometimes the entire abdomen—is distorted. They may occur singly or, as is more common, in clusters—in fact, less than 2 per cent occur singly. (British physician Dr. Victor Bonney has reported removing as many as one hundred fibroid tumors from a single patient!) But they are almost always benign— once removed, they will not grow back. The medical dictionary defines "benign" as "favorable for recovery."

Fibroid tumors constitute the prime reason for the performance of hysterectomy—but, at the same time, those that are severe enough to warrant such radical treatment are in the minority. Most are small enough to be removed independently, and many are simply left alone and observed from time to time. Only the tumors that cause great pain, excessive bleeding, pressure on adjacent organs, or gross distortion of the abdomen indicate removal of the uterus—and the choice is often left up to the patient.

Because fibroid tumors occur primarily in the uteri of

women in the childbearing years and usually regress after the menopause, it is thought that estrogen may have something to do with their growth, although the exact cause has yet to be pinpointed. Recently, investigators have theorized that viruses may be implicated in the growth of tumors, but no one knows for sure. Surprisingly, fibroid tumors occur more frequently in black women than in the Caucasian race, and the reason for this remains obscure.

Though the exact incidence is unknown, gynecologists believe that as many as one of every five women over the age of thirty probably has uterine fibroids. Most of these are too small to be significant, and no treatment is necessary. In fact, it is believed that many women live long and uncomplicated lives with fibroid tumors that they don't even know they have. Of those that require surgical removal, only a small percentage necessitate hysterectomy.

The fibroid tumor usually remains attached to the wall of the uterus. It can develop in the uterus itself, or in the inner wall, or it can expand outside the uterus and into the lower abdomen. When it stays within the uterus, the tumor can remain small or expand into the uterine cavity, causing an enlargement similar to that of pregnancy. Small tumors can remain in the uterus throughout pregnancy and delivery; larger ones may be implicated in cases of sterility and/or habitual spontaneous abortion. In the latter case, their removal can often make possible healthy pregnancies for women who have repeatedly aborted or failed to conceive. Patients should not count on this, however, since many doctors believe that, in some women, the same unknown abnormality may be responsible for both fibroid tumors and sterility.

WHAT ARE THE SYMPTOMS OF FIBROID TUMORS?

Many fibroid tumors occur and exist without symptoms, remaining undiscovered until the patient undergoes a routine checkup. Of course, no one knows how many of these tumors may go undetected in women who are not conscientious about having regular pelvic examinations.

BLEEDING   The primary symptom of fibroid tumor is excessive vaginal bleeding. Often the patient notices that the flow of her normal periods has increased, or the periods may last longer than they normally do. In rare cases, a gushing or hemorrhagic type of bleeding may occur. The fibroid tumor usually will not cause irregular bleeding or spotting, but many other disorders will. In no case should excessive or unusual vaginal bleeding be ignored. After the menopause, any bleeding at all is indicative of some kind of gynecological disorder, and the physician should be called promptly.

In normal menstruation, the uterus contracts at regular intervals to eject a little menstrual fluid at a time and prevent an excessive loss of blood; these contractions cause the "cramps" of which so many women complain. A uterine fibroid, however, can interfere with the normal contraction, allowing the uterus to expel more blood than it should. In such cases, the patient usually begins to notice gradually that she is losing more blood than she normally does, and that her periods are lasting longer, with fewer days in between. Because she is losing too much blood, she is likely to feel exhausted after each period and have difficulty regaining her strength before the next period. Anemia is a common complication in these cases.

Whenever there is a departure from the normal pattern of menstrual bleeding, it is a sign that something is not as it should be. The change is not necessarily attributable to fibroid tumors; in most cases it is caused by something else entirely. But common sense dictates that a gynecologist should be consulted as soon as the unusual bleeding pattern is noticed.

PAIN Most fibroid tumors do not produce pain; when they do, the pain is a sign that complications exist.

Occasionally the fibroid tumor will become twisted within the uterus, to the extent of cutting off its own blood supply (like all organic tissue, the tumor must have a steady supply of nourishing blood in order to exist and grow). When this happens, the tumor begins to degenerate, causing pain and abdominal tenderness.

If the fibroid is sufficiently large, it can press against the upper abdomen, and pain will result from the pressure of the tumor against the stomach and diaphragm. Though most tumors are detected and treated before they can reach such a size, a neglected fibroid tumor can grow large enough to interfere with digestion, elimination, and even breathing.

The large fibroid that extends outside the uterus can also become adherent to other abdominal organs, causing back pain that usually remains constant throughout the month and increases just before the menstrual period. When this happens, the ovaries and Fallopian tubes may become implicated, and it will be necessary to remove them with the tumor.

Because the tumor is a foreign body, the uterus may attempt to expel it by contracting, just as it does in childbirth. The patient who has had children will recognize the resultant pain as identical to that of severe menstrual cramping and labor pains for, in fact, the very same thing is happening. This type of pain will occur intermittently, but almost always becomes worse around the time of the menstrual period.

PRESSURE   The large fibroid tumor may exert pressure against the urinary bladder, the ureter, or the rectum. When the ureter becomes compressed by the bulk and pressure of the tumor, the patient may find it difficult to urinate, and she may feel pain in her back, kidneys, and thighs. Sufficient pressure against the bladder itself can cause actual retention of urine—the patient will not be able to urinate at all, and will have a great deal of pain.

In other cases, the patient who has pressure on her bladder may feel a constant or frequent need to urinate, and find herself running to the bathroom over and over and over again during the course of a day and night.

When the tumor pushes backward against the rectum, constipation results. All of these types of pressure become worse around the time of the period and are particularly pronounced after long periods of standing. The patient who works as a waitress or saleswoman, for example, would probably be more indisposed by this type of pain than would a secretary or executive who spends most of her day sitting.

DETECTION

Because the symptoms of fibroid tumors are, singly and combined, also the symptoms of a number of other disorders, the patient's complaints alone will not zero the physician in on the true nature of the problem. He may first suspect, and investigate, the possibility that something else entirely is causing the pain, bleeding, or abdominal pressure. When he does suspect a fibroid tumor, he will conduct one or all of the following examinations.

ABDOMINAL PALPATION   The word "palpation" comes from the Latin word *palpare*, meaning "to touch." Abdominal palpation is a routine procedure in any general physical examination. With the patient lying on her back, the physician feels the outside of the abdomen with both hands, kneading, pushing, and probing in an effort to detect any abnormalities.

If the fibroid tumor is large enough, it can be felt at abdominal palpation, but a mass felt by the physician is not necessarily a tumor. A swollen uterus, for example, could be merely early pregnancy in a patient of childbearing age. A lump in the area of either ovary could be an ovarian cyst. The small fibroids located in the folds of the myometrium cannot be felt at all in this manner.

Therefore, a diagnosis of fibroid tumor is never made exclusively on the basis of palpation.

PELVIC EXAMINATION   Every woman who has ever visited a gynecologist has experienced this mildly unpleasant type of examination. With one finger in the vagina and another in the rectum, the physician palpates the internal abdomen with a better chance of locating and identifying an abnormality. Even this examination does not positively pinpoint the fibroid tumor, however, since the enlarged uterus or mass could still be mistaken for pregnancy or cysts. It does give the physician a good idea of the size and contour of the mass, and of whether it is tender to the touch.

X RAYS   When he suspects the presence of a fibroid tumor or cluster, the physician may investigate by X irradiation. An injection of an opaque dye into the uterus will cause the fibroids to show up on an ordinary abdominal X-ray picture if they are within the cavity of the uterus.

CURETTAGE   When the diagnosis is not confirmed by X ray, it is often necessary to perform a curettage, a surgical procedure commonly known as a "D and C"—"dilation and curettage."

In this operation, performed in a hospital with the patient under general anesthesia, the surgeon approaches the uterus through the vagina—there is no cutting of the abdominal wall. With the vagina held open by an instrument called a retractor, the cervix is dilated, or opened, and the inner wall of the uterus is gently scraped with an instrument known as a curette. The tissue collected by the curette is then analyzed to determine the nature of its cell structure.

The D and C is a relatively minor operation, performed on hundreds of women each year. It requires only a short stay in the hospital, and postoperative pain is minimal, though the patient will experience bleeding for several days afterward.

TREATMENT

When fibroid tumors are positively identified, and cancer is not implicated, the physician and his patient must decide whether or not to operate.

OBSERVATION If the tumors are small enough, do not appear to be growing significantly, and are not causing the patient to suffer pain, abnormal bleeding, or other distress, the physician often elects simply to leave them alone and hope they will not progress. If the patient is of childbearing age, he must consider her wishes about having children and attempt to determine whether the fibroids are likely to interfere with conception or pregnancy and delivery. If the patient has passed the menopause, the tumors are not likely to change and probably can be left alone. In any case, however, once the diagnosis of fibroid tumor has been established, the patient is instructed to watch carefully for any signs of their progression. Whether or not any noticeable changes occur, she must be examined periodically so that even the most subtle signs of growth can be detected as early as possible.

After the menopause, the fibroid is not only stable in most cases, but may even regress on its own. The regression is thought to have something to do with the fact that estrogen is no longer being produced by the ovaries and that, because of the cessation of menstruation, an adequate blood supply is no longer available to nourish the tumor.

(*Though the following stories are true, all names are fictitious, in respect for the privacy of the patients and their families.*)

Laura C., a single, thirty-four-year-old pediatrician, had put her education and career ahead of romance for most of her life. But she loved children, as her choice of specialty indicates, and when she finally married at thirty-five, she longed to have one of her own. But, a year earlier, trouble had begun.

As a physician, Laura knew the importance of regular

checkups, and had always had a Pap test and physical exam performed once a year by a colleague who was a general practitioner. But when her usually regular periods began to give her quite a bit of trouble, she decided to consult a specialist and chose Dr. B——, a highly respected gynecologist.

After putting Laura through the usual tests, Dr. B—— told her quite frankly that she had fibroid tumors to the extent that she should probably have a hysterectomy. Speaking as doctor to doctor, he was able to present the problem in technical terms with the full understanding of his patient. She realized that, while she *should* have the operation, her fibroids were at that time small enough that a program of observation could be undertaken without danger or too much discomfort.

Most doctors are usually uncomfortable in the role of patient, and Laura was no exception. She felt that, at thirty-four, she was really too young to lose her womb—and, as a doctor, she knew exactly what kind of risk she was taking. So she chose to forego the operation for the time being, and agreed to watch carefully for any changes and to have regular examinations performed by Dr. B——.

During the next year, while Laura's physical condition remained stable, she met and married another doctor and found that marriage had instilled in her a deep desire for motherhood. She decided that she wanted to have a child of her own immediately, while it was still possible—*if* it was still possible. She explained this rather vehemently to Dr. B——, hoping against hope that he would approve of her attempting a pregnancy.

Dr. B—— was skeptical of Laura's chances of conceiving and carrying a pregnancy to full term. Although many women of thirty-five do have babies, the physical strains of pregnancy, labor, and delivery are more trying than they are for younger women. And the complication of the fibroids only magnified the problem. However, knowing that she knew and understood all the medical aspects of the case, including the fact that success was not likely, he agreed that she should try to become pregnant and wished her the best of luck.

Unfortunately, Laura was not to be successful. Though she did become pregnant, she was unable to carry the child to term, and miscarried. By this time, the fibroids had grown to the extent that Dr. B—— practically insisted that she go through with the hysterectomy he recommended.

Naturally, Laura was heartbroken, but took her doctor's advice and had the operation. Physically, she recovered normally, but emotionally she fell into a postoperative depression that hurt both her career and her home life. She was listless and blue, overslept, neglected her normal activities long after her strength had returned, and cried at the drop of an idea.

Laura's reaction was understandable, considering the circumstances—but tragedies occur in every life, and her husband knew that she had to stop feeling sorry for herself and get back to living her life.

With his patience and understanding, Laura slowly began to respond. When it had first been decided that the surgery must be done, he and Dr. B—— had agreed to try to persuade Laura that the answer to the problem was adoption— a suggestion that Laura rejected almost violently in the first grief over the loss of her baby. But, as time went by, her need for a child to love overcame her self-pity, and she agreed.

Though Laura and her husband were older than most applicants for adoption, the fact that they were doctors was heavily in their favor—that and the fact that there are so many children available for adoption these days that the formerly stringent rules have been relaxed in many states. They were successful, and Laura quickly came to love her adopted son as if he had been born to her.

Of course, not all women with fibroid tumors are destined to lose their babies if they are able to conceive. Each case is as individual as the woman to whom it occurs. And Laura's story, like a great many, had a happy ending—despite her hysterectomy.

SURGERY When the patient is still in her childbearing years every attempt is made to avoid hysterectomy unless the patient requests it. Even the woman who already has children and doesn't particularly want more would usually like to preserve her ability to conceive as long as possible, if only for psychological reasons. Therefore, every possibility of removing the fibroid tumors with less radical surgery will be considered. The patient should know, however, that, if the fibroids alone are removed while she is young, there is about a 15 per cent chance of her having to have a hysterectomy or other gynecological surgery later on in life. For an older woman, with removal of the fibroids alone, there is still a slight chance of her having to undergo another bout with surgery.

The primary factors in the decision are the size, location, and rate of growth of the fibroids. If they have been neglected long enough to have filled the uterus, hysterectomy is usually inevitable. In some cases, however, it may be possible to solve the problem with a myomectomy.

Remember that the myometrium is the muscular substance of the uterus. A myoma is any benign neoplasm (new growth of tissue) of the muscular substance of an organ. Thus (remembering also that the suffix *ectomy* means "cutting out"), the meaning of myomectomy is clear: the surgical removal of a segment of the uterine wall.

The decision to perform a myomectomy is based on other factors in addition to the size and number of the fibroids. First, it must be determined that the remainder of the uterus, the tubes and ovaries, and the other abdominal organs are all in healthy condition. This cannot always be determined before the operation, and the patient must be prepared for the possibility that surgery will turn up some condition that will make hysterectomy necessary after all.

The patient's general health must also be considered, as it must in the decision to perform any type of major surgery. If she is grossly overweight or anemic, the operation will probably have to be deferred until these conditions can be corrected.

When the fibroids are removed, the uterus will eventually return to normal. It may be four or five months before it regains its normal shape, but function can usually be restored, depending upon how deep an incision has been made in the uterus and how many fibroids have been taken out. The operation may also mean Cesarean section as a future consideration.

Young patients, even those who have had more than one myomectomy, usually find that it is possible to conceive and go through healthy pregnancies and deliveries after the surgery. In fact, myomectomy may be the factor that permits pregnancy in patients whose fibroids have previously prevented conception or have caused early or habitual abortion.

Myomectomy is also preferred to hysterectomy in the

young woman because it does not necessitate any inter-
ference with the healthy ovaries and their ability to produce
estrogen. For these reasons, myomectomy is the preferred
treatment for fibroid tumors whenever possible.

Karen L., a married woman of twenty-five, had been hoping for a child throughout the four years of her marriage.
Twice she had conceived, and twice she had gone through
the grief of a spontaneous abortion. Suspecting fibroid tumors as the cause of her inability to carry a child to term,
Karen's gynecologist performed all the previously described
tests and determined that she did, indeed, have a small cluster of fibroids on one wall of her uterus.

The doctor told Karen that she would have to make a
difficult but very important decision. She could have a hysterectomy immediately and eliminate all future worry about
the fibroids. However, that freedom from worry might not
be worth the price—the knowledge that she could never
have a baby. On the other hand, the gynecologist could
remove the fibroid tumors alone and take the chance that
Karen might subsequently be able to conceive—but the operation would by no means ensure her ability to become
pregnant. She would then have to live with the possibility
that the tumors might come back—she might have to have
more surgery in the future, and that could include a hysterectomy. He suggested that she discuss the matter seriously
and thoroughly with her husband before deciding which of
two bumpy routes to take.

Because of her youth, and their intense desire to have
children, Karen and her husband elected to take the chance
that a myomectomy might make it possible for her to conceive. Hopefully, she went through the operation.

Many tense and anxious months followed Karen's surgery.

Realistically, she knew that she could not expect to conceive right away, but as each month passed she became more and more nervous and irritable.

The doctor advised her to relax as best she could, explaining that tension and mental anguish can adversely affect the menstrual cycle and also the ability to become pregnant. He also reminded her that the myomectomy had not been any kind of guarantee that she would be able to conceive. As always, it was a *chance*, and he hoped that she had fully understood the possibility that it might not be successful.

Intellectually, of course, Karen did know the facts, but emotionally she found it difficult to accept them, and her nervous state was interfering with every aspect of her life. Her doctor prescribed some tranquilizers and urged her to calm down and find something else on which to concentrate.

Two years after her myomectomy, when she had just about given up hope of ever becoming a mother and had begun working again as a dental technician to keep her mind off her problem, Karen missed a menstrual period. Almost afraid to hope, she saw the gynecologist and happily learned that she was pregnant.

Ecstatic but mindful of her previous abortions, Karen followed her doctor's instructions scrupulously, and eventually was delivered, by Cesarean section, of a daughter. Unfortunately, part of the doctor's prediction did come true—a few years later Karen's fibroid problem returned, and this time there was little choice; she had a hysterectomy. Her relief and joy at being a mother overcame the usual apprehension, however, and Karen regarded herself as lucky to have been able to put the operation off long enough for her child to have been born.

Karen's case is an example of what can—but not necessarily will—happen to a woman who is faced with fibroid tumors while still young enough to be thinking about pregnancy. For older women, however, those who are near, within, or past the menopausal stage, hysterectomy is preferred over myomectomy. Why? Simply because there is always the possibility that additional tumors may grow in a myomectomized uterus, making it necessary for the patient to have to go through another session in the operating room at a later date. Thus, when there is no reason to attempt to prolong the patient's ability to bear children, total removal of the uterus is strongly recommended—and usually preferred by the patient as well as her doctor.

Joanna R., a robust woman of forty-seven, had three children. Most of her life, Joanna had been a housewife, happily spending her days in the prosaic tasks of laundry, house cleaning, and cooking. Yet, when confronted with the fact that she had fibroid tumors, Joanna was terrified. The word "tumor" meant "cancer" to her, and she feared that she was faced with an early death, leaving her children with only their father to care for them.

Joanna's fear is not uncommon—magazine articles, movies, and television plays have led many people to think that the word "tumor" is always synonymous with cancer. But such need not be the case, for there are many kinds of tumors that are not cancerous; fibroids are among them.

When Joanna first noticed irregularity in her menstrual periods, she attributed it to the fact that she was nearing the age of menopause, and assumed that it was just one of the "female troubles" she would have to endure as she went through the "change of life." But when her periods became noticeably longer rather than shorter, she became concerned. Too, as her periods lengthened, Joanna noticed that her energy had begun to ebb. While she was by nature an active person, she now felt exhausted much of the time, virtually gave up the golf and horseback riding that she loved so much, and found herself taking naps several times a day. Finally, after several months of distress, Joanna consulted her gynecologist, Dr. G——.

From his patient's complaints, Dr. G—— immediately suspected that she had fibroid tumors, but he couldn't be sure until he had performed a very thorough examination.

Abdominal palpation told him nothing, so he performed a pelvic examination (which he would have done anyway—abdominal palpation is not a conclusive procedure, but sometimes gives the doctor a further hint of what to expect).

The pelvic examination revealed that Joanna's uterus was enlarged—and it was unlikely that she was pregnant because she had been very faithfully taking her birth-control pills. Too, Joanna's age indicated that, while pregnancy was certainly not impossible, that and the fact of her profuse bleeding made it most improbable.

By this time, Dr. G—— was pretty sure that Joanna's problems were being caused by fibroid tumors—but he wasn't positive, and no ethical doctor will recommend costly and traumatic surgery on such flimsy evidence. He asked Joanna to undergo X-ray examination, and she agreed—even though, by this time, the idea of cancer had inevitably occurred to her, and she was frankly quite afraid of what the examination would reveal.

Dr. G—— injected opaque dye into Joanna's uterus, then took the X rays. The pictures convinced him that fibroid tumors were, indeed, the root of her troubles. At this point, he and Joanna together had to decide what to do about them—and several factors of her case would influence the decision.

First, Joanna was very close to the age of normal menopause, and could expect to lose her childbearing ability
within the next few years, no matter what. Second, she already had three children, all in their teens, and had no
desire for a new baby. On the basis of these facts, Dr. G——
recommended that Joanna undergo a hysterectomy. He told
her, frankly, that he did *not* think she had cancer, but that,
considering her age and the fact that she had children, a
hysterectomy would be the safest course—if left alone, the
fibroid tumors could grow and cause her a great deal of distress.

Nevertheless, Joanna was severely frightened. After several months of anxiety, she consulted her husband, telling
him that she feared the hysterectomy was the only way to
save her life.

Unfortunately, Joanna unwittingly transmitted her own
panic to her husband—but, at the same time, her fears
caused him to agree that she should have the operation. Together, they made the right decision for the wrong reason,
since Joanna's life was not threatened by her fibroid tumors.

After the surgery, Joanna and her husband made a very
good adjustment. To her own surprise, she felt no less feminine, but Dr. G—— assured her that it was no surprise to
him since femininity is based in the mind rather than the
uterus.

Other patients with fibroid tumors have been less fortunate than Joanna. Some, though not many, are young and
childless. But Joanna's case is pretty typical—and the decision that she and her husband made was in their own best
interests. Left alone, Joanna's fibroids could have grown to
the point of causing her pain and disfigurement. In cases
such as hers, any decision is a gamble—but the patient and

her husband would be wise to allow themselves to be guided by the experienced physician's advice, since only he or she knows the true odds.

After the menopause, fibroid tumors usually regress; if they are not discovered until that late in life, chances are that they are insignificant and can be left alone. If they do cause symptoms or show signs of growing, however, hysterectomy is preferred to myomectomy for the reasons previously stated.

ENDOMETRIOSIS

It would be a mistake to think that a diagnosis of endometriosis automatically dooms a woman to losing her womb. In fact, this disease is one of the less common indications for hysterectomy, and can usually be treated by less radical means.

The word comes from *endometrium,* the mucous membrane that lines the inner surface of the uterus, and the suffix *osis,* which means "a process." Therefore, it would be natural to assume that endometriosis is a process that goes on in the endometrium. But this is not always true, and the literal translation of the word is misleading. Endometriosis occurs most frequently in the ovaries and can crop up anywhere in the abdomen. In rare instances, it has been found in such remote places as the lung and thigh.

Endometriosis is a collective term used to describe growths, often called implants or cysts (but not all cysts are endometriosis, so we shall call them implants). The tissue that makes up these implants closely resembles the normal endometrial tissue; hence, the name.

The implants react to the normal hormonal cycle as does the true endometrium; for this reason, the disease almost always occurs during the reproductive years. It has been found in only a few teen-aged girls and postmenopausal women and, after the menopause, it is a sign that hormonal stimulation still exists. By far the greatest incidence is between the ages of twenty and fifty, and the majority of these patients are between thirty and forty.

Often, endometriosis will occur concomitantly with other disorders. Whereas almost two thirds of patients with endometriosis experience irregular bleeding, less than 20 per cent of these women have endometriosis alone; most also have fibroid tumors or polyps in the uterus.

The incidence of endometriosis has increased significantly over the last thirty years, during which time there has been a trend toward delaying childbirth until later in life. The disease has always been much more common in the high-income groups, in which birth control is more prevalent and childbearing is often saved for after the early years of marriage. It is known that women in the lower economic and educational groups have more babies earlier in life than do the college-educated and well-to-do, and the younger and more prolific mothers are statistically less likely to contract endometriosis. Also, endometriosis is thought to be associated with infertility, either early in life or during the later childbearing years. For these reasons, it has been postulated that early and frequent pregnancy may do something to the abdominal organs that prevents the formation of the abnormal implants; it's possible, but no one is sure. Certainly no woman should make a point of getting pregnant early and frequently in the hope of preventing this disease; the population explosion is a far more serious problem.

Endometriosis is most often found in the ovaries and on the inner surface of the uterus, and it occasionally occurs in the Fallopian tubes, intestines, bladder, and appendix. It is thought that the disease may, in some instances, be prompted by surgery, since the implants are sometimes found in the scar tissue of a healed incision or on the stumps of amputated organs.

When endometriosis occurs in the ovaries, the implants are usually known as "chocolate cysts," because they contain a thick brown fluid, or old blood. Once started, the chocolate cyst is most likely to grow with each menstrual period, and will eventually have to be removed. Their removal does not always entail hysterectomy, however. Often it is only necessary to remove a portion of the single affected ovary, and the uterus and other ovary will remain intact.

When the implants remain in the uterus, they will look, at first, like little blue pimples or powder-burn stains. Like the chocolate cysts, however, they grow larger each month, and may bunch together to produce firm, hard nodules. If left untreated, they can grow large enough to spread into the vagina, cervix, and surrounding abdominal tissue.

SYMPTOMS

PAIN   By far the most common symptom of endometriosis is menstrual pain, which many women dismiss as "cramps." But, as the disease progresses, the pain will become steadily worse with each period and take on a dull, heavy feeling. The pain usually begins just before the period, getting worse and worse until the actual flow begins, then slacks off during the next few days of bleeding. By the end of the period the pain has usually stopped. But it will recur with the next period, getting worse each month, until the woman finally consults her doctor. If she has never had this kind of pain before, and is over twenty-five years of age, chances are good that the diagnosis will be endometriosis.

As the endometriosis grows, it may also cause severe backaches or pain at the time of sexual intercourse. If it has spread backward toward the rectum or forward toward the bladder, the patient may begin to notice increasingly painful elimination. Occasionally the implants will spread into the intestines, in which cases there may be severe intestinal cramps.

INFERTILITY   Technically, we cannot say that infertility is a true symptom of endometriosis since failure to conceive can be caused by so many other factors, including male sterility. But it is true that about 40 per cent of patients with proven endometriosis have difficulty in becoming pregnant, and the remainder usually do not have large families. No definite reason for this has been established, but it has been noted that many patients with endometriosis have anovulatory cycles, that is, cycles in which no egg is released by the ovary. This occurs when the implants are located in the ovaries. If the ovaries are not affected, ovulation still occurs, but fertilization seems to be inhibited, in many women, by the disease process. It is also thought that the pain of intercourse that often accompanies endometriosis may cause the woman to reduce her sexual activity, thereby lessening her chances for pregnancy.

BLEEDING   Though many patients with endometriosis have abnormal menstrual periods, the irregular bleeding is not thought to be a direct result of the disease. It is much more probably caused by some sort of malfunction of the ovaries, such as sclerosis, or hardening, of the capsules that enclose the ovaries.

DETECTION

PALPATION   When the gynecologist suspects that his patient has endometriosis, he will first perform a pelvic examination. With one finger in the vagina and another in the rectum, he will palpate, or feel, for lesions on the pelvic organs. When he finds them, both he and the patient will know it, for the implants of endometriosis are very tender to the touch, and the examination will be painful. He will also probably find that the uterus has moved backward from its normal position and is slanted upward rather than tipped forward; it is likely to be immovable from this position.

These findings, while characteristic of endometriosis, also indicate associated diseases, such as pelvic inflammation and fibroid tumors. So the diagnosis of endometriosis cannot be made on the basis of palpation alone.

CULDOSCOPY AND LAPAROSCOPY   These are ten-dollar words that describe a process by which the gynecologist can look directly at the internal pelvic organs. To do this he uses an instrument called an endoscope (*endo*="within"+"scope"="an instrument for examining"). In culdoscopy, the endoscope is inserted deeply through the vagina, and the physician peers through his end to see what he can see. The examination is not particularly pleasant, but if it can enable the doctor to detect early endometriosis, it is well worth the temporary discomfort it may cause. Laparoscopy, performed with the same sort of instrument, is a penetration into the abdomen, through the wall of the abdomen at or near the navel.

Other methods of detection will be used if it is suspected that endometriosis exists in other parts of the body, but, since they are not concerned with hysterectomy, they will not be described here.

TREATMENT

The treatment of endometriosis depends upon the extent of the disease and upon the location of the implants. For our purposes, we shall be concerned only with those that arise in the reproductive organs.

Because most of the patients are still in their childbearing years, every effort is made to treat endometriosis by some method other than hysterectomy. Each patient is an individual, of course, and the physician must take into consideration her age and her desire to have a child. If she is older and already has all the children she wants, the prospect of hysterectomy may not seem quite so grim, but it will probably still symbolize a loss of youth and femininity.

OBSERVATION In some cases, when the patient is young, the pain is slight, and the extent of the endometriosis appears to be minimal the patient can be left untreated and observed from time to time. Many women would prefer to put up with their pain and try for pregnancy before any kind of treatment is begun.

MEDICATION It has been found that the growth of the implants regresses sharply if the patient can manage to become pregnant, or when the ovaries fail to release their eggs. When menstruation stops at menopause, so does the spread of the disease. Therefore, it is sometimes possible to retard or even reverse the growth of the endometriosis with the use of hormonal drugs that inhibit ovulation.

These are, in many cases, the same drugs that are used for birth control—the highly controversial "Pill." When a woman is pregnant, the amounts of estrogen and progesterone in her body are increased. These "pregnancy levels," among their other functions, prevent the ovaries from releasing eggs during the pregnancy. Thus, when pills are taken to raise the nonpregnant woman's hormonal levels to the amounts present during pregnancy, ovulation will not take place.

When the pills are taken for birth control, the patient stops taking the drug for a few days each month to allow normal menstruation to occur. This is done because the endometrium builds up normally during the month despite the ovulation-inhibiting effects of the drug, and should be allowed to flow out at the end of the cycle. However, when the medication is prescribed for the treatment of endometriosis, the patient will be instructed to continue taking the pills for an uninterrupted period of time determined by the doctor—sometimes as long as six months. During this time the endometrial implants will usually shrink and sometimes even disappear, though this result cannot be counted upon. The pain should become milder or disappear altogether, and the chances of a successful pregnancy will, hopefully, be increased.

There has been a great deal of publicity about this sort of treatment lately, with the medication usually being called "fertility drugs." Though the reasons for these regimens include various conditions other than endometriosis, many women have been treated successfully for infertility in this manner, since use of the drugs regulates the menstrual cycle, enabling a couple to more accurately determine the best time to attempt conception. On the other hand, the drugs have also been blamed for multiple births, most notably the famous Kienast quintuplets. When used for birth control, they have been held responsible for blood clots and even cancer. Some doctors say that the dangers of taking hormonal drugs are less than the dangers of going through a normal pregnancy; others believe these drugs are too dangerous to be used.

In any case, the decision for or against hormone therapy will depend upon the individual doctor, and the patient would be wise to discuss the matter with him at great length —particularly if she has been trying unsuccessfully to have children.

In some cases the male hormone, androgen, has been used to inhibit ovulation because it is thoroughly effective in doing so. But it has its price: It has been found to have masculinizing effects. Some patients who have taken androgens have experienced characteristics common to adolescent boys—hair grows on their faces, they break out in acne, and their voices begin to crack and become deeper. For these reasons, androgens are not widely used by women.

Whether or not hormonal therapy is used, the doctor will probably prescribe some kind of medication to relieve the pain associated with endometriosis—and the type of drug will depend upon the individual patient.

SURGERY If hormonal treatment fails—or if it is considered worthless or dangerous in a particular instance—surgery will usually have to be performed. Unless the patient is one of the few postmenopausal women who have endometriosis, every effort will be made to preserve her ability to have children, or her ovarian function if she wants no more children.

If it is at all possible, the surgeon will remove only the actual implants, leaving most of the uterus and ovaries. If the ovaries and the tubes are affected, he will try to save at least one set of them, and this can often be done. There is always the risk that some invasive tissue will be left behind and that the disease will recur, but most doctors believe that the risk is well worth it when the patient wants to have children.

Only when this kind of conservative surgery is impossible, or fails, will the gynecologist and surgeon resort to hysterectomy.

CHAPTER 4

Why Hysterectomy Is Performed:
Cervical Cancer and Endometrial Cancer

"CANCER" IS A VOLATILE WORD. To the astrologically minded, it signifies people born between June 22 and July 22—but even many astrologists have changed the name of this category to "Moon Children" because of the disease connotation.

In Webster's Dictionary, cancer is, among other things, "a malignant evil that corrodes slowly and fatally." That's a bit strong, for though cancer is malignant, it is not necessarily slow or fatal. "Malignant," incidentally, means, "tending to go from bad to worse"—cancer does not just sit there, it must be caught in its natural act of deadly progression and, when possible, stopped.

In Dorland's Medical Dictionary, cancer is "a cellular tumor, the natural course of which is fatal and usually associated with the formation of secondary tumors." This, too, is slightly misleading, since *treated* cancer is no longer always fatal. Once all cancer was—and to this day we do not know how to prevent it—but, through early detection, surgery, and irradiation, physicians have found ways to keep it from killing.

Cancer can attack any organ in the body, and as some of its causes, investigators have cited air and water pollution, cigarettes, and the chemicals with which our "modern" foods are treated. But none of these is implicated in the cancer with which we are concerned: the cancers of the female reproductive system.

CANCER OF THE CERVIX

The cervix of any organ is its neck, or a necklike part. The uterine cervix, then, is the narrow lower portion that opens into the vagina (see Chapter Two). Any part of the cervix can become infiltrated by cancer, but the lesions are usually located on the outer surface that can be seen through the vagina (*Figure 2*).

Happily, statistics show that the incidence of death caused by cervical cancer has declined steadily in recent years. For this, much credit must be given to the organizations and communications media that have so well educated the public about the importance of early detection and treatment. Also, new techniques have been developed to aid the physician in spotting abnormalities as quickly as possible. As more and more women learn the importance of regular examinations, the incidence of death—and hysterectomy—attributable to cervical cancer should become negligible.

The incidence statistics also yield some surprising information implicating factors that would seem to have no bearing on an individual's susceptibility to a given disease.

For example, the incidence of cervical cancer among women of the religions in which baby boys are circumcised

—notably the Jewish and Mohammedan—is about one-ninth that among women of other religions. Apparently, this can only mean that *non*circumcision is in some way connected with cancer, though no one is quite sure why. Of course, this cannot be considered the sole factor, since cancer does occur among Jewish women married to Jewish men and among women of other religions whose husbands just happen to be circumcised. But their chances of avoiding it seem to be more favorable.

Race is also an apparent factor, with cervical cancer occurring more frequently in the nonwhite population. The exact reason for this has not been documented in scientific terms, nor has any genetic evidence been found to indicate that any one race "carries" or is physiologically "predisposed" to this form of cancer. But the socioeconomic correlation is obvious, and the deplorable living conditions under which the whites still force so many members of minority races to exist are clearly incriminated as being contributory. In any community in which opportunities for good hygiene are poor and access to adequate medical care is limited, the incidence figures will be higher in any category of disease—particularly one whose proper care demands early discovery. Physiologically, no gynecological differences among the races have ever been documented.

It is probably also true that the age of first sexual contact and the frequency of intercourse are very important. Doctors generally believe that the greater the frequency and the earlier the age of first intercourse, the greater is the chance of cervical cancer.

Mothers of large families are more susceptible to cervical cancer than are those with few children, and the woman who has never given birth is safer yet. Again, the reasons are not known, but, since the disease has been linked to physical irritation of the cervical tissue, the probabilities are clear.

For the same reasons, frequent sexual activity appears to heighten a woman's chances of acquiring this disease, even if she remained a virgin until relatively late in life. Statistics show that women who practice sexual intercourse regularly are more likely to fall victim to cervical cancer than are those whose sexual activity is rare.

All of this sounds terribly discouraging. It begins to look as though one might as well become a nun. However, nuns and secular women who are proven virgins have been known to have cervical cancer. The incidence is low, but it does happen. Obviously, then, something besides (or in addition to) sex and childbearing is behind the development of this disorder. When someone finally discovers what it is, perhaps we can focus most of the blame on that and retire happily to our bedrooms with lighter hearts.

Of course, cancer is not the only disease that can affect the uterine cervix, and it is a mistake to panic when an examination turns up a lesion or infection. Most of these can be treated—and should be right away, since nonmalignant cervical irritations may be precursors to cancer if they are neglected.

Whenever a cervical disorder is detected, the gynecologist will take a sample of the tissue for a microscopic study. Often, merely a smear of the vaginal mucus is sufficient; or it may be necessary to cut out a tiny piece of the cervical tissue, called a biopsy specimen. In most cases, these samples will prove to be benign; when they are not, rapid treatment may be enough to prevent the need for major surgery. Occasionally, however, when the lesion has been neglected or gone undetected for some time, hysterectomy will become necessary.

WHAT ARE THE SYMPTOMS?

BLEEDING   As is the case with fibroid tumors, bleeding is the primary symptom, but the bleeding caused by cervical cancer is of a different nature.

This type of bleeding is most commonly called spotting. Rather than having an excessive or irregular flow, the patient may notice episodes of very sparse bleeding in between her normal periods. This slight bleeding may be brought on by some sort of jolting activity such as horseback riding, jogging, or driving over a bumpy road. Most frequently it is noticed after sexual intercourse.

Noticed, yes, but often dismissed. The amount is so slight, and the episodes of spotting so irregular, that the patient is likely to think of them as nothing, and not bother to have them investigated. This could be a serious error, since cervical cancer is the most common cause of this type of bleeding —not the only one, but certainly the one that should be investigated the most quickly. As has been stated, any kind of irregularity in menstruation is a danger signal deserving swift action.

VAGINAL DISCHARGE   The discharge caused by cervical cancer may be odorous. This discharge will be watery and range in color from yellowish-white to brown. It usually begins about the same time as the spotting.

PAIN   The early cervical cancer does not cause pain. The only symptoms are the bleeding and slight discharge, both of which are innocuous. When there is pain, it can only mean that the disease is in an advanced stage, in which case the bleeding and the discharge will have increased to such a degree that they can no longer be ignored.

Once the disease has reached this stage, however, it is often too late for effective treatment. The pain indicates that the disease has spread to dangerous proportions.

There cannot be too much emphasis placed on the importance of checking out even the most subtle changes in the normal pattern of bleeding. The most inflexible rule in any kind of uterine disorder is to catch it early—it could be a matter of life and death.

DETECTION

When the gynecologist suspects cervical cancer, he will first perform a pelvic examination, though this method of diagnosis is only conclusive if the disease is far enough advanced to be felt and/or seen.

If the patient consults her physician as soon as she notices any of the previously described symptoms, the cancer will often be so small as to be undetectable to touch or to the naked eye. As part of the pelvic examination, the physician will then take what is known as a "smear," or a sample of the vaginal mucus surrounding the cervix. This examination is painless, and is done with either a slim suction tube or a cotton swab. The material obtained is smeared on a glass slide and sent to a laboratory for analysis. It is usually several days before the results are obtained. This test, called a "Pap smear," is a routine part of every pelvic examination and is done in the hope of catching any cancerous development even before it has progressed enough to cause symptoms.

If the smear results are negative, other possible reasons for the patient's complaints will be investigated. If the results are positive, further tests will be made. The diagnosis of cancer cannot be made solely on the basis of the vaginal smear, since there are some women whose smears will indicate cancer when actually none exists.

BIOPSY The word biopsy is a combination of *bio,* meaning "life," and the Greek *opsis,* meaning "to see." The biopsy, then, is a minor operation that permits the diagnostician to see, under the microscope, what is going on in living tissue.

Before the biopsy of the cervix is done, a test will be performed that will hopefully point out the exact site of the cancer; this is known as the Schiller test, after the physician who devised it.

With the patient in the pelvic examination position, the gynecologist will stretch the vagina open with a vaginal speculum. With a cotton swab on the end of a slim forceps, he will cleanse the surface of the cervix and then paint it with a liquid known as Schiller's solution; this consists of iodine, potassium oxide, and water. It causes no pain.

When the cervix is painted, its normal tissue will be stained a dark, mahogany brown. If the cancerous area is on the outer surface, it will not take the stain and will remain pink, pinpointing the spot from which the biopsy specimen should be taken. It is possible, though, that the cancerous cells may be located beneath the surface tissue or far enough inside the cervix that they will not show up. In such cases, a greater number of specimens will have to be taken. The primary purpose of this test is to locate as closely as possible the area to be biopsied.

The biopsy is a simple procedure, performed without anesthesia in the physician's office. There is no pain, because the nerve endings in the cervix react painfully only to stretching. With the vagina again held open by a speculum, the physician uses an instrument called a punch biopsy forceps to nip off several small specimens from the area indicated by the Schiller stain. (If the Schiller tests did not indicate the area of cancer, specimens will be taken from all around the cervix.) There is very little bleeding, and what there is can almost always be controlled by the application of a small wad of cotton.

Some physicians prefer to locate the biopsy site with a colposcope, an operating microscope that enlarges the view of a specimen to thirteen times its actual size.

The biopsy specimens are then analyzed microscopically in an effort to disprove the diagnosis of cancer, or to confirm it and determine the nature of the disease.

SURGICAL CONIZATION   Occasionally, even the biopsy specimens do not provide enough accurate information. In such cases the patient must be hospitalized so that a cone-shaped segment of cervical tissue can be removed for analysis. This operation, though relatively uncomplicated, is nevertheless much more extensive than the simple biopsy, and is performed with the patient under general anesthesia. There is more bleeding, and the patient should expect to stay in the hospital for about three days after the operation.

TREATMENT

Cancer is a disease about which scientists have put forth many hypotheses but have not found any universal solutions. The tumors appear to be as individual as the patients

—and as unpredictable. There have been women with barely discernable cancers who have deteriorated rapidly, and there have been others with massive cancers who have lived actively for years without treatment. Of course, these are the extremes, and most cases fall in between. But it should be understood that there is no hard-and-fast rule that can be applied to every patient, and treatment can be established only after the gynecologist has performed a number of tests in hopes of selecting the best method for the individual patient.

The final choice of therapy is based on a number of factors: the extent of the cancer, the patient's age and general condition, and whether or not there are additional abdominal disorders to contend with.

When cervical cancer is discovered in a pregnant woman, the method of treatment depends both upon the extent of the disease and upon the length of the pregnancy. If the malignancy is not discovered until the latter part of pregnancy, attempts will usually be made to wait until the baby can survive outside the uterus. Then a Cesarean-section birth will be carried out along with a hysterectomy, followed by radiation therapy—obviously, the radiation cannot be started during pregnancy because of possible damage to the baby. If the cancer is discovered early in pregnancy, however, it is almost never believed safe to wait; therapeutic abortion and hysterectomy are performed, and radiation is instituted shortly thereafter.

The plight of the expectant mother who must both lose her baby and face the dread fact of cancer is sad, indeed. But she must also bear in mind that the physician's prime concern is for her life.

Marcia G. and her husband both loved children and were

looking forward to having a large family—a hope that they were sure they had begun to realize when her first pregnancy was confirmed.

As every pregnant woman should, Marcia kept regular appointments with her obstetrician for prenatal examinations. But, late in her pregnancy, Dr. M—— detected what he was sure was an early carcinoma (cancer) of the cervix. The doctor believed that a hysterectomy was the only treatment that would save Marcia's life. He urged Marcia to allow him to terminate her pregnancy and remove her uterus—but, determined to have at least one child of her own, Marcia refused, knowing that surgery cannot legally be performed without the patient's written consent.

Marcia became so distraught that her husband insisted that she see a psychiatrist. She did, only to learn that this doctor, too, believed she should undergo the operation despite the shock of losing both her child and the hope of ever having any others of her own.

Still she refused, stubbornly rejecting the efforts of friends, family members, and doctors to persuade her to be sensible. She became very nervous and upset, cried a great deal, and made life generally miserable for herself and all the people who loved her.

Close to term, Marcia went into premature labor. Rushed to the hospital in pain and mental anguish, she was finally able to accept the fact of the inevitable and signed the form that would give the doctors permission to perform a hysterectomy if her lesion proved to be the malignant disease that her doctor suspected.

Unfortunately, it did. Marcia's baby was stillborn, and a hysterectomy was performed at the time of delivery.

When she regained consciousness and learned what had

happened, Marcia was near emotional collapse. Like many women, she had always believed that her prime role in life was that of a mother, and once robbed of her ability to produce children of her own, she felt useless and thought that life was not worth living.

Long sessions with the psychiatrist, as well as the love and support of her husband, family, and friends, eventually convinced Marcia that pregnancy and childbirth are actually only a prologue to the role of mother and the greatest accomplishment of a maternal woman lies in her ability to *raise* children, to give them love, and to guide their lives. She could waste her life moping and feeling sorry for herself, or she could enrich the lives of several adopted children by directing her maternal instincts to their benefit and raising them as she would her own.

Fortunately, Marcia recovered from her depression and became a loving adoptive mother to four children; her husband, too, loved them with the dedication of a natural father.

Rather than allow herself to be conquered by an unavoidable obstacle, Marcia learned to put the unfortunate experience behind her and devote her life to carrying out her original ambition. She succeeded in achieving her goal despite having had to take a side step along the way.

RADIATION Radiation is preferred by some physicians to surgery—as is any alternative to hysterectomy. But there are some patients on whom it is useless. Although the radiation is intended to kill the cancerous cells and destroy the invaded tissue, some tumors are found to be resistant—that is, they remain unaffected and continue to grow. In other cases, failure of radiation therapy can be blamed on the nature not of the cancer itself but of the surrounding normal tissue, called the host.

When radiation is decided upon, the method to be used depends, again, upon the individual case. Some patients are hospitalized, and undergo implantation of tube-shaped radiation applicators inside the uterus, cervix, or vagina. In some cases, irradiated platinum nodules are inserted directly into the cancerous tissue. Other women can be treated on an outpatient basis, reporting to the radiologist's office several times a week for external application of X rays. This is tedious, and some patients experience undesirable reactions to the procedure.

When radiation therapy has to be discontinued, it is not always because of ineffectiveness. Occasionally, complications may occur, usually in the form of a lowered white blood cell count or radiation sickness. The latter consists of nausea and vomiting, and is an indication that the dosage is too high, or that the treatments are being given too often.

Though these complications are a potential hazard of radiation therapy, the physician is well aware of them, and the method and frequency of application are carefully chosen accordingly.

SURGERY   Unfortunately, unlike the fibroid tumor, cervical cancer does not lend itself to an alternate method of surgical treatment; when surgery is decided upon, it is hysterectomy. The type of hysterectomy that is chosen (the different types will be described in a later chapter) is usually the radical type that includes the removal of the adjacent lymph nodes. This will once again depend upon the extent and nature of the disease, the patient's age and general condition, and, in this case, her weight. The heavier a patient, the more difficult it is for the surgeon to operate.

Obviously, when radiation can do the job without endangering the patient in any way, it will be the chosen method of treatment. But if complications arise that cannot be remedied by changes in the type, amount, or frequency of radiation, the patient will have to resign herself to the fact that hysterectomy is inevitable.

CANCER OF THE ENDOMETRIUM

As we have pointed out, the endometrium is the mucous membrane that lines the inner surface of the uterus. The word comes from two more Greek words: *endo,* meaning "within," and *metra,* meaning "in relationship to the uterus." Thus, the endometrium fits the definition by being within the uterus and in direct relationship to it, and is, in fact, part of it.

About 75 per cent of the women who get endometrial cancer are past the menopause, which occurs, on the average, between the ages of forty-eight and fifty. In general, the term "postmenopausal" can usually be taken as meaning "over fifty." (There have been women who have conceived and borne children after the age of fifty, but they are rare.) Only 10 per cent of endometrial cancer patients are between the ages of twenty and forty, and 15 per cent are between forty and fifty.

Endometrial cancer is much less dangerous to life than is cervical cancer, and there is a higher overall cure rate. This type of cancer spreads much more slowly, and is often limited to the actual body of the uterus.

This very confinement, however, makes it much more difficult to detect, since it cannot be seen and often cannot be felt. The vaginal smear does not always signal its presence, and its symptoms are shared by a number of other uterine disorders. Postmenopausal bleeding is often the first clue.

In recent decades there has been a noticeable increase in the incidence of endometrial cancer, probably because more women are living until the late years in which it usually occurs. Unlike fibroid tumors and cervical cancer, endometrial cancer is rare in the black race—and no one has the answer to this puzzle. It is suspected that the higher birth rate among black women may have some significance, since endometrial cancer more often affects the woman who has never been pregnant, whereas cervical cancer usually strikes the woman who has borne children.

Suspected as the principal cause of this disorder (though no one specific cause has yet been pinned down) is an excess of estrogen production after the controlling effects of the other female hormone, progesterone, have ceased because of menopause. Both human case histories and laboratory studies on animals have implicated this possibility but, again, endometrial cancer has occurred in women who do not appear to have any such hormonal imbalance. Like all forms of cancer, it remains a mystery, constantly studied in hopes of an eventual breakthrough.

Although there are, of course, exceptions, a pattern has emerged that seems to fit the majority of women who contract this disease. Though it certainly cannot be said that all women who fit this description will fall victim to endometrial cancer, it has been noted that a significant number of patients will fit into one or more (usually more) of the following categories:

LATE MENOPAUSE   Though the menopause usually occurs at about age forty-eight to fifty, many patients with endometrial cancer do not begin to stop menstruating until about six years later. It has been theorized that the six extra years of estrogen production may have something to do with the development of the cancer.

HEREDITY Approximately 20 per cent of patients come from families in which there is a history of cancer. Although this leaves 80 per cent who have no such family history, the figure is considered statistically significant by physicians.

OBESITY Although a great many women gain weight during and after the menopause, most endometrial cancer patients have been overweight during youth and middle age. This kind of obesity is not the ordinary consequence of overeating, however, but is the result of some kind of hormonal imbalance (some people who blame their fat on "glands" aren't just making excuses). There is a specific body build that is implicated, in which the patient has a stocky frame, small hands and feet, and heavy, bulging hips.

OTHER DISORDERS The endometrial cancer patient is very likely to also have hypertension, that is, high blood pressure (about 50 per cent of patients do), and may also have diabetes (about 15 to 20 per cent have it, and nearly 50 per cent show positive reactions to the test) or arthritis. These diseases, too, are often attributed to improper hormonal levels, suggesting that the endometrial cancer may be simply another result of the imbalance of hormones. It must be stressed, however, that the existence of these conditions is not necessarily a forewarning that endometrial cancer is on the way. Many women with hormonal imbalances live their entire lives without ever having any kind of cancer. But the woman who does fit this clinical pattern will be wise to have frequent gynecological checkups, particularly after the menopause.

PREGNANCY AND CHILDBIRTH Unlike the cervical variety, endometrial cancer tends to occur more frequently among women who have had trouble getting pregnant, have had one or more miscarriages, or have only one child. Not many of these patients have many children, a fact that can be theoretically attributed to the same hormonal imbalance that is thought to eventually produce the cancer. This theory is disputed, but some doctors do suspect that the fact that so many endometrial cancer patients have had trouble conceiving and delivering may be an indication that something has been wrong inside the uterus all along.

Excessive production of estrogen is fairly generally accepted as a cause of endometrial cancer, yet it is not thought to be solely to blame. Although there are probably factors that have not yet even come under suspicion, it is thought that the overabundance of estrogen may merely condition the uterus in some way that will eventually make it a suitable host for the cancer. In support of this theory are records showing that a great many endometrial cancer patients have previously been discovered to have what is known as uterine hyperplasia—an excessive growth of the normal endometrial tissue. The word comes from *hyper,* meaning "excessive," and *plasia,* meaning "formation." It is, in simple terms, an overgrowth of the uterine lining. Because this condition is found in so many women who later have endometrial cancer, it is thought that the excessive growth of tissue may create an environment favorable to the later invasion of the cancer.

If we accept, for the moment, the excessive estrogen theory—and today most doctors do—we must then try to determine what causes the ovaries to produce more of this hormone than they should. As with most medical questions, there is no one, sure answer, and there may be many reasons as yet undiscovered. It is thought, however, that some malady of the controlling glands—the adrenal and pituitary—may be at fault. Ovarian tumors have also been blamed in many instances, as have the estrogen replacement drugs that many gynecologists prescribe for women going through and past the menopause. Hopefully, these synthetic hormones will lessen the incidence of hot flashes and masculine characteristics that are often produced by the menopausal loss of estrogen. Opinions vary as to whether or not this type of therapy can lead to cancer, however, although there is no conclusive evidence that it does.

SYMPTOMS

VAGINAL BLEEDING Cancer of all types is still surrounded by hundreds of "maybes" and "what ifs" and theories. But one definite statement can be made: After the menopause, any kind of vaginal bleeding, of any nature and amount, is cause for immediate investigation. In many cases it will *not* be caused by cancer. But to ignore it is to play very foolish games with one's life.

Bleeding is the most important and most frequent symptom of endometrial cancer, particularly when the patient is —as most are—past the menopause. In the young woman it will appear as irregularity of the periods or as spotting in between the normal bleeding times. The periods will usually last longer than they should, and the patient will probably notice a significant increase in the quantity of the flow. This kind of bleeding is most often found to be caused by something other than cancer—such as fibroid tumors—but it cannot be overlooked.

The spotting type of bleeding is not at all uniform in character or amount. Unlike the bleeding of cervical cancer, it will not usually occur after sexual intercourse, but is likely to appear when the patient is straining at stool. This kind of spotting can occur whether the patient is one of the few young women who contract endometrial cancer or is past the menopause. Among postmenopausal patients, however, 10 per cent of the women who experience bleeding turn out to have endometrial cancer. Though slight spotting is the most common type of postmenopausal bleeding, some patients experience a sudden, gushing type.

VAGINAL DISCHARGE In many cases of endometrial cancer, the patient will notice a clear, watery discharge even before the onset of irregular bleeding. If disregarded, the discharge, which may be preceded by cramps, will change gradually to a brownish hue. It may eventually take on a foul odor.

PAIN Pain may or may not occur, and cannot be accurately described as a symptom of endometrial cancer; many patients experience no pain at all. When it does occur, it is usually described as a feeling of pressure rather than as a definite pain.

DETECTION

The chief obstacle to both detection and treatment of endometrial cancer is that it cannot be seen and, in many cases, cannot be felt. This leaves the physician relying on the vaginal smear, endometrial biopsy, and curettage.

VAGINAL SMEAR This technique is only a preliminary when endometrial cancer is suspected. While a positive result to the test is significant, a negative result cannot be trusted, since the cancer may be located far up in the uterus and not discard cells into the vaginal fluid.

ENDOMETRIAL BIOPSY This is performed in the same manner as is a cervical biopsy (Chapter Four, page 51), except that the cervix is dilated to allow the surgeon to reach inside the uterus with the punch biopsy forceps and collect specimens from the endometrium.

CURETTAGE This procedure is the only trustworthy method of detecting endometrial cancer, and should be performed on any patient who reports bleeding after the menopause. Unfortunately, a number of women are reluctant to go through with it, for a variety of reasons. As has been described, the lining of the uterus will be scraped, and the collected tissue will be examined microscopically. Occasionally, however, even this technique can fail to disclose a small cancer concealed in an out-of-the-way part of the uterus. If the postmenopausal patient continues to bleed after her first curettage has yielded negative results, the operation will have to be repeated.

TREATMENT

Most physicians prefer total hysterectomy, after a period of preparatory radiation, as the one best method of treating endometrial cancer. Though there are a few who believe that radiation alone is the most effective and safest therapy, most physicians will not use it in place of the operation unless the patient is considered unfit for surgery. If she has diabetes or hypertension to an extensive degree, there is too much danger in subjecting her to the stress of surgery. Also, a patient who is very old and feeble or very fat will be deemed ineligible. In such cases, a program of radiation will constitute the sole therapy.

RADIATION External radiation (X ray) treatment may be effective when the patient is not too fat. When she is, the intensity necessary to be effective on the cancer would be so strong as to be damaging to the skin. In most such cases, radium capsules are implanted in the uterus through the cervix.

MEDICATION Progestational and chemotherapeutic agents are also used when the patient is unfit for surgery, but they are a second choice and subject the patient to the possibility of having to endure a wide range of side effects that may or may not accompany a treatment that may or may not be effective.

SURGERY The decision as to whether or not surgery should be performed depends upon the grade of malignancy and the size of the uterus. When it is warranted, the accepted operative treatment for endometrial cancer is total hysterectomy, preceded by radium treatment. The removal must be total, and include the removal of both ovaries and tubes, so that no cancerous tissue is left behind to begin growing again. Most doctors prefer to delay the operation until after a thorough course of radiation, in an attempt to kill as much of the malignant tissue as possible and to reduce the size of the tumor. When radiation is not performed prior to surgery (and it is omitted only in selected cases), there is a much greater chance that some living cancerous tissue may be left behind, or that the operation itself may implant such tissue in a previously unaffected part of the vagina or lower abdomen.

Though surgery of this sort is traumatic at any age, it is considered fortunate that endometrial cancer strikes mainly after the menopause, when a woman is no longer concerned about having children. When the patient is a young woman, the anguish of losing her womb can only be balanced against the far greater anguish of possibly losing her life.

CHAPTER 5

Must the Ovaries Go?

UNFORTUNATELY, MANY PEOPLE, both women and men, equate hysterectomy with complete loss of feminine function. The reproductive function is, of course, lost with the removal of the uterus; however, as has been mentioned previously, the secondary sex characteristics of the female exist with or without the presence of that organ. Those traits include enlarged breasts, lack of facial hair, the characteristic female figure, and voice tone that is higher in pitch than that of the male.

None of these is controlled or even influenced by the uterus; that organ is there merely to provide a favorable environment for the monthly ovum, to nourish and house the embryo and fetus after the ovum is fertilized, and to dispose of its soft inner lining when the ovum is not fertilized. The balance of femininity is determined in two ways: physically by the ovaries and their hormones—estrogen and progesterone—and mentally or psychologically by the mind and emotions of the individual patient.

In this chapter, we are concerned only with the physical properties of femininity. Every woman has heard of the menopause, the often-dreaded "change of life," and all can expect to experience it if they live past the reproductive years. Hysterectomy, however, brings to many the fear of "instant menopause," though this need be true in only a small percentage of cases—those that necessitate removal of both ovaries as well as the uterus. Often the ovaries can be saved and will continue to secrete estrogen (see Chapter Two) as long as they remain viable—that is, until they must be removed at a later operation, or until they cease to function through natural menopause.

Let us emphasize that the ovaries do not degenerate after the surgical removal of the uterus.

Every organ in the body is kept alive and working by a continuous supply of blood. The ovaries, though they work with the uterus in creating a child, are separate organs that receive their life-sustaining supply of blood from two sources: 1) from the uterine artery, and 2) from an artery called the infundibulo-pelvic artery. When the uterus is removed, the utero-ovarian artery is closed off, but the blood supply to the ovaries (which maintains their viability and productivity of estrogen) remains intact through the infundibulo-pelvic *ligaments,* which contain the blood vessels that lead directly to the ovaries (*Figure 2*).

Thus, the ovaries do not shrivel and die when the uterus is removed, nor do they even slack off in their production of estrogen as far as we know. *The estrogen supply remains essentially the same as long as the ovaries are intact.*

Happily, the same statement holds true in those cases in which one ovary must be removed; in these cases there are no adverse effects, nor is there any alteration in ovarian activity.

Nature has provided the human body with several sets of

duplicate organs, such as the lungs and kidneys, and most of us have heard of cases in which one of these had to be removed for one reason or another—for example, the case of actor John Wayne, who has lived with characteristic vigor for many years with one lung, since the other had to be surgically removed because of cancer. When a diseased organ of one of these sets is removed, its partner continues to function as long as it remains healthy. Thus, removal of one organ of a pair does not seriously compromise the other's normal function, nor the well-being of the patient. So it is with the ovaries.

Even when the uterus is perfectly healthy, many women must undergo removal of one ovary because of the presence of a cyst or other disease. As long as the other ovary and the uterus remain in good health, such women will still be able to anticipate motherhood because the remaining ovary will be capable of taking over the job of providing ova for possible fertilization as well as that of maintaining the secondary sexual characteristics.

In some cases, one ovary can be left behind even when the other must be removed with the uterus, a situation that can be brought about by a condition known as "ectopic pregnancy." Christine F. had just such a problem. At the age of twenty-six, several years after the birth of her daughter, Christine became pregnant again. At first her doctor was puzzled: Though Christine had missed a period by the time she consulted him, he was unable to detect the usual enlargement of the uterus that would have indicated pregnancy.

Further examination disclosed the fact that Christine had an infrequent but not unknown problem: The ovum, once fertilized in the Fallopian tube, had, for some unknown reason, been unable to make its normal journey into the uterus and had become embedded in the wall of the Fallopian tube—ectopic pregnancy. If the condition had not been detected as early as it was, the embryo would have continued to grow there until the tube could no longer contain it and would have burst—a condition that, if not properly treated, could have caused the mother's death from blood loss.

Fortunately, Christine had sought medical help early, as should all women who suspect that they are pregnant. She underwent an operation that necessitated the removal of the tube in which the embryo was growing (and the embryo itself, of course) as well as her uterus. Such an operation may also be necessary when the embryo is embedded in the cone of the uterus—the junction of Fallopian tube and uterus. In such a case, the problem is known as "cornual pregnancy."

After her operation, Christine was depressed about the loss of her baby, her uterus, and her ovary, and feared the worst. Though she was able to accept her inability to bear any more children, and was grateful that she had one of her own, she dreaded the thought that she might become an "old woman" at an early age.

Christine's doctor assured her that her fears were groundless and that her remaining ovary would continue to provide her body with as much estrogen as she would need until the onset of her natural menopause. She would never again have a period, of course, because she had no uterus. However, the doctor explained, she had one child and was still every bit a woman in every way except for the ability to bear another. And she need never fear an unwanted pregnancy, take another birth-control pill, or have to wear a diaphragm or intrauterine device. She had, in effect, built-in birth control.

Though Christine was a bit dubious at first, time proved her doctor to have been right. She remained exactly the same gynecologically, except for the loss of her ability to conceive and the elimination of monthly periods. If trouble had occurred later with her remaining ovary (which it didn't and was not likely to), it would have had no connection with the loss of her uterus and first ovary.

Occasionally, the title of the chapter must be answered, "Yes." There are cases in which both ovaries must be removed along with the uterus and, when the patient is premenopausal, this does bring about the rapid onset of symptoms associated with the "change of life." Such a procedure is done, however, only when physicians consider it essential for the preservation of the patient's life and/or well-being, or for the prevention of further difficulties, as in the case of Diane (Chapter Eight).

Why must both ovaries go? There are a number of reasons. For example, any serious infection of the ovaries that would compromise their integrity—such conditions include tubo-ovarian abscess, an infection that affects both tubes and both ovaries and produces severe pain. Another is postabortal gas gangrene of the uterus—such conditions make it important that both ovaries be taken out, as would a chronic, severe inflammatory disease of the pelvis.

Tuberculosis, a disease thought by many to be restricted to the lungs, can be spread through the bloodstream to the ovaries and may make it necessary that they be removed.

When a young patient is discovered to have cancer of the breast, surgical removal of both ovaries is often recommended to control the spread of the disease when it has lodged in other places. (The medical term for such an operation is "oophorectomy," pronounced "oh-oh-for-ectomy.")

When the patient who must have her uterus removed is more than forty years of age, many physicians recommend that both ovaries be removed simultaneously as a matter of course. This is strictly a preventive measure, based on the knowledge that cancer of the ovary has suddenly assumed major proportions as a killer of American women. Though the reason is still unknown, and probably will be until this dread disease is finally conquered, physicians find more cancer of the ovary now than ever before, and the incidence of its developing in a patient who has had a previous hysterectomy is considerable.

In the December 1974 issue of *Ca—A Cancer Journal for Clinicians,* strong statistical evidence to back up this belief is presented by Drs. Hugh R. K. Barber, Edward A. Graber, and Tae Hae Kwon, all of Lenox Hill Hospital in New York City. Their studies have shown that close to half (46.7 per cent) of the deaths caused by gynecologic cancer are directly attributable to malignancy in the ovaries. The disease is expected to affect ten of every thousand American women over the age of forty, and of these ten, only one or two will be saved. Further, close to 10 per cent of those patients who have ovarian cancer have previously had their uteri removed *without* excision of the ovaries. The doctors believe that routine preventive removal of the ovaries along with the cancerous uteri could prevent a significant number of deaths among these patients.

Stating that "The ovary may get too old to function, but it is never too old to form tumors," the doctors point out that most ovarian cancer occurs in women between the ages of forty and sixty-five. Thus, when a woman of that age must have a hysterectomy for cancer affecting her uterus or cervix, concurrent removal of the ovaries makes a great deal of sense in terms of her future health and, indeed, her life expectancy.

For this reason, a number of physicians have assumed the attitude that both ovaries should automatically be removed at the time of hysterectomy if the patient is nearing the age of natural menopause. Most doctors, however, will disagree with the all-inclusive term "automatically," preferring to treat each case on a strictly individual basis.

Once it has been determined that both ovaries must be removed along with the uterus, what can the patient expect? If she has already experienced her menopause, nothing; once the discomforts of surgery have receded, she will feel, physically, the same as she did before her operation. If the patient is young, however, she will have to accept the fact that menopausal symptoms will occur very much sooner than she had expected them—probably within several days to a week after surgery.

These symptoms will probably include hot flashes, a condition in which the patient feels suddenly very hot for a few minutes or seconds and then returns to normal temperature; weight gain; depression; a thinning of the bones, a condition known as osteoporosis; sometimes touches of arthritis; and sometimes a change in her sexual appetite, which varies with the individual—some women desire more sexual activity, some less. The appearance of aging should not be accelerated beyond the rate at which it would normally occur, but this cannot be documented because there have never been any controlled studies done on the subject.

Though these sound like dire predictions, the picture is

not as gloomy as it may seem. No premenopausal hysterectomy patient need fear all of the previously mentioned
conditions any more than she can expect to escape them all;
the incidence is as individual as the patient. But, whatever
difficulties ensue as the result of premature ovarian loss,
they can be treated.

At present, the treatment known as "estrogen replacement" is still controversial. While some doctors swear by it,
others continue to condemn it, and still others sway from
side to side as the debate goes on. The prevalent opinion
seems to be that, if menopausal symptoms begin, estrogen
replacement may be begun while the patient is still in the
hospital and should be continued thereafter. Such therapy,
administered properly, will most probably delay the menopausal changes after oophorectomy, and these benefits may
be continued for many years.

Why, then, do some doctors object to it? Although this
has never been proven, there are those who think estrogen
replacement may hasten the occurrence of breast cancer or
cause weight gain and fluid retention. Though this is a
theory, it is enough to deter some doctors from prescribing a
treatment that is known to be highly beneficial in many
women. Sometimes, too, the patient may find that her
breasts are a bit more tender to the touch than usual.

On the positive side, in addition to virtually eliminating
premature menopausal symptoms in an impressive number
of patients, estrogen replacement causes the vagina to retain
its normal degree of lubrication—very important to sexual
intercourse. One of the many complaints of patients going
through the natural menopause is that dryness of the vagina
makes intercourse uncomfortable and often even painful.

It is also believed that estrogen replacement helps to retard the onset of degenerative vascular disease; that is, disorders of the body's fine system of veins. Taken together, the advantages seem to heavily outweigh the possible disadvantages when such important treatment is being considered, especially when the patient is still young.

Just what is estrogen replacement? It is exactly what the term implies: replacement of the estrogen production that has ceased through the loss of the ovaries, whether that loss be by surgery or by Nature (menopause). Thus, estrogen replacement given to premenopausal patients who have had their ovaries removed is essentially the same as that given to women who have gone through the natural menopause.

Estrogen replacement is usually given in the form of pills, though occasionally injections are used. The pills or injections contain various concentrations of synthetic or natural estrogens that assume the functions of the estrogens that have been lost. In most cases, after examining the patient, the physician will, with full knowledge of her past history, write a prescription that can be filled at her local drug store. Occasionally, he may administer an injection and then either ask her to return at regular intervals for additional shots or prescribe pills that can be taken at home to maintain the needed level of the hormone. In any case, he will recommend that she make periodic appointments for further examination, and the wise patient will keep them scrupulously.

In most cases, the estrogen that is given a patient postoperatively or postmenopausally is very effective in counteracting the uncomfortable results of estrogen loss and will maintain her in a state of good health, free from hot flashes, weight gain, irritability, depressions, and so forth.

Again, it must be stressed that each patient is unique unto

herself. Estrogen replacement must not be regarded as a miracle cure for her ills. But neither hysterectomy nor menopause need be thought of as the end of life as a woman; both physically and mentally, a woman is a woman is a woman—and can and should be for the rest of her life.

CHAPTER 6

Who Has a Hysterectomy?

THOUGH A GREAT MANY WOMEN are unfortunate enough to have the disorders described in the previous chapters, not all will have to go through with a hysterectomy. In deciding whether or not to operate—or how extensively to operate— the gynecologist and surgeon must take a number of factors into consideration.

We already know that cancer is one of the reasons that the operation must be performed—it is just too risky to take a chance on the patient's losing her life. And there are other situations that will prompt the physician to tell his patient that she *must* undergo hysterectomy, giving her very little choice in the matter.

BLEEDING

One of these is excessive uterine bleeding, which may occur in a pregnant or nonpregnant woman. Depending on the underlying cause, in many instances there may be no way to control a constant and heavy flow other than per- formance of this type of operative procedure. To the woman, this kind of bleeding may seem merely an irritant, or a source of constant bother—certainly nothing so serious as to warrant going through an operation! But the physician knows otherwise—that a continual loss of blood from any source is a vitally serious matter. It can cause the patient to become weak and anemic, sap her strength, and even threaten her life. If surgery is the only way to stop such bleeding, then surgery it must be.

INFECTION

A serious infection is another indication for mandatory hysterectomy. The type of infection that can follow abortion (much more common in the days before abortion was legalized in the United States) or a very severe pelvic inflammatory disease can occasionally result in death unless a hysterectomy is performed. Of course, not all infections are this serious, and the evaluation of each one's gravity can only be made by the doctor.

ADJUNCTIVE SURGERY

Occasionally when a surgeon is performing an operation for removal of a malignancy in the ovaries, or even in the lower intestinal tract, he may find that the uterus must be sacrificed as part of the operative procedure. This type of unexpected hysterectomy will be quite a shock to the patient who awakens to find that her uterus is missing when all she expected to lose was a tumor of an ovary or a bit of intestine. But she must realize that a surgeon is often surprised by what he finds when he looks inside the body, and anything that threatens the life of the patient will have to be taken out. Obviously, the surgeon is the only one qualified to make that decision, a fact the patient acknowledges when she signs the papers that give him permission to operate.

The surgeon's prime concern regarding any organ in the body is his patient's ultimate welfare. Will she survive and maintain or regain a condition of well-being if the organ in question is left in the body? The same problem is posed by the surgeon who removes a kidney, a lung, or a gall bladder, and the final decision must rest with him. In most cases, however, the surgeon who is faced with removing a uterus when he did not anticipate doing so will consult with several of his colleagues before proceeding with the surgery. Only when a consensus of learned opinion determines that retention of the diseased uterus would endanger the patient's life will the doctor perform an unplanned hysterectomy.

PHYSICAL OBSTACLES

When the nature of the disease does not make hysterectomy a life-or-death procedure, there are still a number of other considerations that go into the physician's decision for or against operation.

WEIGHT One serious consideration is the patient's weight. If she is within normal limits for her height and build, then of course no problem exists. If she is excessively thin, then the reason for her lack of weight may be significant, though the thinness itself will not interfere with surgery. But why is she so thin? The answer could be a disease process such as tuberculosis, or it could be directly attributable to a malignancy of the uterus or some other organ. In such a situation, the patient's blood volume is markedly diminished, and she may have to go through a number of blood transfusions before or after surgery, or both.

The worst weight problem, of course, is obesity. There is no surgeon who is happy about operating on a fat patient. All the possible complications of any surgery—bleeding, postoperative infections, respiratory problems with anesthesia—are much more likely to occur among fat patients than among those who are relatively slender. If the patient needs to have a hysterectomy, however, obesity *per se* will not stand in the physician's way of making the suitable decision. Often, if a patient is obese and the uterus is not too large, a vaginal operation can be done, eliminating the necessity for an abdominal incision and its consequent problems.

It is important to point out, however, that the very obesity itself may be a part of the *cause* of the problem that has made the hysterectomy necessary. Many patients who have cancers in the body of the uterus are fat—and physicians believe that the excessive weight may well be a precipitating factor. It is known, for example, that women who have diabetes, obesity, hypertension (high blood pressure), and no children are much more likely to have cancer of the uterus than are those who do not have this combination of predisposing factors.

The moral, as usual, is that people should not allow themselves to get fat, a dictum that should surprise no one. Many other diseases, affecting men as well as women, can be traced to excessive weight—the most notable among these is heart disease, which kills even more people than does cancer. "Stay slim" is good advice to anyone.

DISEASE CONDITIONS   Often, the patient who seems to be a candidate for hysterectomy may have other diseases that constitute problems to the surgeon. Some examples are heart disease, blood disorders, respiratory infections or other diseases (tuberculosis, emphysema, etc.), or associated infections. Heart disease can usually be handled without too much difficulty unless the patient is very seriously compromised, and such disease, in itself, seldom stands in the way of a hysterectomy. Actually, if the woman is very seriously disabled by a disease of her heart, chances are that the heart condition will be responsible for her death before any uterine disease has a chance to manifest itself.

Patients with serious heart problems of long duration usually do not live to the age at which gynecological problems that call for hysterectomy are likely to appear. Conversely, acute heart problems (those that occur suddenly, such as heart attacks) seldom happen to women until quite late in life—long after the age at which hysterectomies are usually performed. Therefore, hysterectomy and heart disease are not likely to be simultaneous considerations.

Emphysema (a lung disease that makes it difficult for the patient to exhale, or breathe out), unless it is so severe that the woman is unable to manage on her own, should not be a problem. The choice of anesthetic may be different from the usual types that are used—the anesthetist may choose a spinal injection rather than inhaled gas—but this will not interfere with the operation. The patient who has emphysema and is told she must have a hysterectomy need not worry that her lung disease will make the surgery dangerous.

The same is true of the diabetic—diabetes, a disease brought about by some patients' inability to balance the amount of sugar in the body, can occasionally be aggravated by the shock of surgery. But, since the patient will be in the hospital and under constant care both before and after the operation, her blood sugar will be carefully monitored and her medications regulated according to the orders of the doctor who regularly treats her diabetic condition.

Diseases of the blood, such as leukemia or the several disorders that can cause excessive bleeding, can be a very important consideration when contemplating any kind of surgery. They are so rare, however, that they really do not warrant the time it would take to describe them. Any woman who has one of these diseases will have had a lifetime of treatment, and should she eventually need a hysterectomy, her specialized doctors will have the situation well in hand.

Severe infections, of the type that may or may not be related to the pelvis, may cause the postponement of a hysterectomy but will not stand in the way of its eventual performance. Such infections can interfere with both the anesthesia and the actual surgery. If the patient has pneumonia, severe hepatitis, or pancreatitis, for example, the surgeon will choose, if he possbily can, to put off any surgical procedure until the illness is well under control and the patient is back to normal.

Of course, all of the foregoing are physical considerations that the physician has to take into account in deciding who should have a hysterectomy and who should not. Emotional considerations are something else entirely, since they are completely individual and completely unpredictable.

THE LIFE SITUATION

Even when a patient is in good general health (aside from her gynecological problem) and therefore a prime candidate for hysterectomy, there are occasionally extenuating circumstances that require thoughtful evaluation.

MOTHERHOOD OR NOT? Foremost among these is the patient's desire to have children, which depends, to a large degree, upon her age. If she is twenty-five and childless, for example, the gynecologist will be much less likely to opt for hysterectomy than he would be if faced with a forty-five-year-old grandmother. The rule of thumb among physicians is: If a woman wants to have children in the future, every effort will be made to preserve her ability to do so. The hysterectomy will be put off if at all possible, and the doctor will attempt to successfully remove whatever the causative factor may be—a fibroid, a premalignant cancer of the cervix, or even a possible malignancy of one ovary when the other ovary is healthy and can be spared. It can be said without any reservation that, if the uterus can be saved without endangering the hopeful mother's life, the uterus will be saved.

Whatever is chosen for a patient who wants to have children, the physician will have to make a selection among various courses of treatment that will allow her to maintain her childbearing potential—unless she is on the brink of death, and patients young enough to have babies are almost never in such dire straits.

Unless there is a truly severe disease, such as life-threatening cancer, menstrual bleeding so excessive as to cause anemia, or a disease that in itself prevents the bearing of children (severely damaged Fallopian tubes or ovaries damaged by an infection), some other means of treating her disease will be undertaken until she has had as many children as she wants and can have.

On the other hand, it is often the sad fact that the disease for which the doctor needs to operate is sufficiently severe as to interfere with the patient's childbearing function. It may not totally eliminate the possibility, but may complicate matters to such an extent that childbearing is virtually impossible. When this occurs, it is indeed a tragedy for the patient, but one she must learn to overcome—hopefully, when all chance of childbearing is gone, she will be able to find happiness in adopting and caring for one of the many homeless children who are so much in need of the love she has to give.

Today, with circumstances vastly improved for women in almost every area of life, and choices of life-style becoming more varied and free of the traditional taboos of centuries, many women are finding (and finally being able to admit, even to themselves) that they don't *want* children. Others will find it far easier than ever before to adjust to childlessness and discover avenues of endeavor never before open to them.

Ever since the Suffragettes obtained the vote, women have been emerging from the cocoon of home-and-motherhood that for so long comprised the only *acceptable* mode of life ("spinsters," after all, were once to be pitied even if virtuous, and "career women" were considered either harlots or homosexuals). Now, when the surgeon who performs the hysterectomy may very well be a "fellow" woman, the patient who loses her uterus can either adopt children or adopt the attitude that, with the career of motherhood scratched, she still has a wide-open field from which to choose an alternative.

IDENTITY CRISIS   Another important factor in the doctor's decision is the woman's *desire* to retain her uterus, even when she has no desire for more children—or any children. Regardless of its childbearing function, the uterus is thought of by many women as being the center of their identities as females. The idea of losing it is, to them, tantamount to losing their femininity, and they will protest most vigorously against the operation.

Far too many women remain convinced that the removal of the uterus will result in (1) a change in physical appearance; (2) a radical and undesirable shift in weight; or (3) a deterioration in sexual performance. Although these possibilities are at best remote after a hysterectomy and have no medical basis at all, any woman can bring them about merely by believing strongly enough that they are inevitable. This type of reaction, of course, is not exclusive to hysterectomy or even gynecology—the power of the mind can create all sorts of disorders for which there are no physical causes. Both the patient and the doctor have to contend with the patient's fears about what will happen after surgery—and the more realistic the patient can be, the better off she will be.

THE FACE IS A MIRROR   If she insists on being despondent, overdramatic, and melancholy, there will, indeed, be a change in the posthysterectomy patient's physical appearance—she will look just as haggard as she has let (or made) herself feel. Worry and depression can create wrinkles around the eyes and mouth even in young women; frown lines between the eyes can add years to any face; and the cumulative effect over weeks and months can be devastating.

Vitality, on the other hand, is equally obvious in the face, and with no effort at all on the part of that face's owner. The woman who rejects boredom and laziness in favor of an active interest in life, living, and doing—through her existing career, a new career, a civic activity or charity, politics, an artistic endeavor, volunteer work, travel, return to the care of an already established family, pursuit of a new man, whatever—is automatically going to look as alive as she feels.

More than ever, the posthysterectomy patient should keep herself from becoming self-centered—and that, of course, is most easily done by centering her attentions on other people and outside activities. "I'm bored with being bored," many hospital patients say—and what a healthy outlook that is!

The patient who can look upon her hysterectomy as a gift of life and begin to really *live* that life need not be concerned about her physical appearance. Her face will reflect her inner feelings, and her spirit will show in her eyes.

THE WEIGHT'S THE SAME   As for weight, that, too, is up to the patient. A sound diet and the right amount of exercise will yield proper poundage, period—hysterectomy or no hysterectomy.

The patient who uses her operation as an excuse to eat or drink too much of the wrong things is only compounding a problem that was of her own making in the first place—self-indulgence as a result of self-pity. Too many people eat compulsively whenever their lives are upset by any disturbing event. Food—or in some cases, drink—becomes a pacifier, and they gobble the goodies until they are fat, ugly, and at least twice as miserable.

However, *there is no physical relationship between the uterus and metabolism* (the process by which food is converted to either energy or fat). When both ovaries are removed, the resultant sudden change in hormonal balance may increase some women's *tendencies* to gain weight, but that can be controlled by a proper food intake, high in protein (meat, fish, cheese) and low in starches (sugar, candy, pastry).

Coupled with the right amount of exercise for the individual's physique and capacity (and the capacity will increase as the postoperative period lengthens and strength returns), good eating habits can only produce the right weight for each body. Under no circumstances will a hysterectomy alone cause a patient to gain weight—she has to do that to herself.

A HAPPY LOVE LIFE   Sexual gratification, as will be explained, is in no way affected by the surgical removal of the uterus. It is, however, extremely susceptible to fluctuations in a patient's mood or psyche.

All the nerve endings that provide erotic stimulation and pleasure are located outside and away from the uterus and ovaries. Removal of the uterus, even with the cervix, in no way distorts the anatomy so as to make intercourse impossible or even difficult.

If the patient complains that her vagina has "dried up" after the operation, her physician will either prescribe estrogen replacement therapy (if removal of the ovaries has caused a change in hormonal balance) or suggest the use of a lubricating cream or jelly or estrogenic vaginal cream. Otherwise, there should be no change at all for either the patient or her partner—if the man is someone she met after her surgery, he need never even know about it unless she chooses to tell him!

Appearance, weight, sex—all can be just as they were before the hysterectomy—or, in many instances, better!

Nonetheless, whether a woman is twenty-five, forty-five, or sixty-five, if she insists upon retaining her uterus in spite of a condition that the doctor believes warrants removal, she should do it with an understanding of the risks involved.

There really can be no hard and fast rules regarding a patient's treatment—in the last analysis, the decision will be up to the individual patient and her individual doctor—but it is the duty of the physician to educate the patient as clearly as possible as to just what the problem is and what is likely to happen if his advice is followed—or if it is not.

FEAR AND FEMININITY   A patient's emotions are often very difficult for the doctor to assess. There are those who should have an operative procedure but refuse it because they are either frightened or feel that a hysterectomy would compromise their femininity. Because most gynecologists and most surgeons are still men, they are often somewhat bewildered by a patient's reluctance to "be sensible" and have the operation for practical reasons, casting aside her anxieties as if they didn't exist.

Although the doctors know that such anxieties are unfounded, and that no loss of femininity will occur unless the patient herself brings it about, to the patient the fears are sometimes so burdensome as to be debilitating and blot out all ability to reason. Such patients can, if not dissuaded and cajoled by sympathetic and understanding physicians, relatives, and friends, make heartbreakingly sad decisions that will adversely affect not only their own lives, but those of the people who love and are closest to them.

For example, there was Jenny, who saw her doctor with a complaint of excessive menstrual bleeding. An examination revealed that Jenny had fibroid tumors and should have a hysterectomy in order to conserve her blood—she was anemic, and her condition became worse every time she menstruated. Her doctor reasoned that Jenny, at the age of forty, probably had about ten years to go before the menopause would finally control her bleeding—ten years in which she should be able to lead an active, happy life with her husband and growing children. A hysterectomy would enable her to have those ten years without the distress of excessive bleeding and the weakness brought about by the resultant anemia.

But Jenny's disease was not immediately life-threatening, and she was afraid of the surgery. A hysterectomy, she thought, would make her less a woman, less attractive to her husband, less motherly to her children. She didn't want any more children, so that was no problem, but still—she just didn't want to lose the part of her that, in her mind, made her a woman. Jenny refused to have the operation.

Jenny's doctor found himself in the position of having to make a compromise. His patient's life was not in danger, so he could not feel justified in insisting she go through with the surgery he recommended. And he knew from experience that trying to badger her or scare her into giving her consent might easily make her more adamant and stubborn than ever.

But the doctor knew that she would continue to be ill,

continue to be uncomfortable and incapacitated if she rejected the necessary surgery because of an unrealistic fear. He explained, carefully, what life would be like for her if she tried to manage without the help of the hysterectomy, but still Jenny resisted. She could manage, she insisted, if only she didn't have to lose her uterus.

Jenny's doctor did the only thing he could do under these difficult circumstances: He prescribed iron tablets to try to stem the loss of energy she suffered each month as she expelled more and more blood.

Jenny's course progressed as her doctor had predicted it would—she did not die, but she was virtually incapacitated for seven to ten days each month. When she could, she walked around—but pale and anemic, really unable to enjoy life as a woman in her forties should. Most of the time she was tired, too tired to join in the activities her husband and children enjoyed. She was not a total invalid, but she was hardly the buoyant companion or enthusiastic sexual partner her husband remembered her as having been before her disease had struck. Fearing the loss of her femininity, Jenny had instead lost her vivacity through her refusal to have the operation that would have spared her fatigue and anemia.

Her physician was rueful about Jenny's case. "It's much like having a patient who has an ulcer," he told her husband. "This patient has severe pain from the ulcer. He can't eat, he can't sleep, he can't do much of anything normally, he's just in misery. And yet his decision against surgery can spur his ulcer on. The operation is something that may not be absolutely necessary to save his life, but it would certainly improve his state of well-being."

In Jenny's type of case, as in that of the ulcer patient, it is not the place of the doctor to act as a salesman, to insist that a patient do something she does not want to do, but to give her the best advice he can—to spell out the advantages and disadvantages, and hope that she makes the right choice.

Unfortunately, communication in this respect can be very difficult. There are some patients with whom the doctor can discuss the problem thoroughly; there are others who will listen to absolutely nothing. Not only won't they listen, but often they will seem to listen, but actually be practicing "selective hearing." They hear what they want to hear, and simply will not comprehend what they don't want to admit is real.

In the long run, it is not worthwhile to either the doctor or the patient to continue to discuss the problem time and time again when the patient has made up her mind against following the doctor's advice.

The intelligent patient will listen and come to understand just what the ramifications of an operative procedure are— and what is almost certain to occur if surgery is refused— and then make a calculated decision as to what she prefers, hopefully with her own best interests in mind. Often, patients choose to see one or two other doctors who may, with advice usually approximating that of the original physician, help them to crystallize their feelings about the matter.

Family members, too, can be important influences, either helping or hindering a confused and frightened patient in making her decision. This is a particularly important consideration in some ethnic and religious groups.

Maria J., for example, came from an extremely large and close family in which important decisions were never left up to one member alone. When told that she should have a hysterectomy, her feelings were ambiguous—she did not want to go through with the surgery, but she certainly did not want to risk death or prolonged illness by refusing it. Seeking to have older and wiser heads make the decision for her, she went first to those members of her family who were considered the leaders—her great-uncle and great-aunt, who had pioneered the family's emigration to America. Since Maria had already had as many children as were considered necessary, the elderly relatives advised her to go ahead with the operation, in the best interests of her health.

Though discouraged by their advice, because she did not want to lose her uterus, Maria accepted it. But she did not stop there. Hoping to find dissension that would provide the basis for an argument, she turned to her parents. They, too, agreed that a mother of four had no more use for a uterus that was diseased and making her ill. Finally, under pressure from her family, Maria underwent the operation and was spared years of discomfort and illness.

Not all patients are so fortunate as to have understanding families. Some, finding disagreement within the family ranks, will use that disagreement as an excuse to put off surgery until their symptoms become so severe that they must give in in order to obtain relief. Often, a patient who is close to her family will seize upon one dissenting opinion and cling to it as a good reason for avoiding the necessary surgery. Such women are merely escaping, and eventually find themselves paying for their escape with pain, incapacity, and long-lasting illness.

WHAT ELSE TO DO?

When the physician decides, for one reason or another, that his patient is not a good candidate for hysterectomy, or when the patient out-and-out refuses to have the operation, what are the alternatives? Unfortunately, they are relatively few and far between. External application of radiation and radium, though still used occasionally, have for the most part been eliminated as being poor second choices to surgery, and hormonal therapy has come under a great deal of criticism recently—much more so *before* surgery than after.

Of course, there are other kinds of surgery that can be employed when the condition is not serious enough to warrant removal of the entire uterus. But when a hysterectomy is really needed and is refused, all the doctor can do is try to make his patient as comfortable as possible with medications, knowing that there is no way for her to avoid going through the grief he knows will ensue.

When the problem is excessive bleeding, hormones can often help, although they should not be counted on as a solution. With male hormones and certain female ones, it is possible to stop the type of excessive bleeding that is called hyperplasia, or functional bleeding. There are disadvantages, however—the male hormones tend to masculinize a woman, sometimes causing her to grow facial hair and experience a deepening of her voice. Her upper arms and torso may become chunky, losing their feminine contours. How ironic for this to happen to a woman who rejected hysterectomy because she thought it would rob her of her femininity!

Female hormones, on the other hand, though frequently helpful *after* surgery, are no substitute for the operation when the diseased condition remains. In certain individuals, they may cause an increase in weight through fluid retention (this is not the same as weight-gain caused by overeating), and they are occasionally responsible for nausea and certain allergic reactions. Nevertheless, if a patient really desires to remain on hormones for a long period of time, this type of therapy may bring her some relief if her disease is amenable to it.

When the excessive bleeding is functional and is not connected with any kind of blood abnormality, one of two types of hormonal programs can be used. First, a combination of estrogen and progestin, the same combination that makes up the birth-control pills, will lessen the quantity of the menstrual fluid if the patient has hyperplasia or if she fails to ovulate. Second, excessive bleeding from fibroid tumors can occasionally (but not always) be controlled by the use of progestins.

Testosterone, a male hormone, can sometimes be helpful, but must be used with great caution since it often causes enlargement of the fibroids and induces them to grow at a really rapid rate. Doctors have not been able to reach a universal agreement on this subject—some think the progestins are contraindicated in the presence of fibroid tumors—so the treatment that the individual patient receives will depend on how her particular physician feels about these drugs.

With so few alternatives when a hysterectomy is really called for, the projected consequences of rejecting the surgery are usually pretty grim and can range anywhere from severe compromise to eventual death.

Barbara, for example, was a woman in her sixties whose doctor was convinced that she had a uterine malignancy. At her age, what reason could there be for preserving the uterus? Nonetheless, when the doctor advised a hysterectomy, Barbara refused. She left the hospital, had a minimal amount of X-ray therapy, and began to suffer from a spread of the tumor. Philosophically, Barbara rationalized her problem by saying, "I'm going to die of something fairly soon anyway, so I may as well die of the cancer." In such a case, of course, there is nothing the physician can do but try to ease his patient's discomfort and help her to die as easily as possible. She made her choice, and that was that.

In all fairness, it must be pointed out that the situation is not always that bad. Physicians are as human as anyone else, and their decisions are not (at least not yet) based on mathematical accuracy. And the human body has fooled the best of them. Everyone has, at one time or another, heard a doctor say, "I simply can't understand why that patient is still alive—she should have died years ago." This is true, too, of the conditions that call for hysterectomy.

The wise patient, however, will follow her physician's advice, particularly when it is reinforced by the opinions of his consultants. Self-treatment is so risky that even doctors themselves shun it. The patient may go through all kinds of agonizing and doubt, but when surgery is urged by one or more physicians of high qualification and reputation, she will serve only her best interests by allowing herself to trust them and do as they say, allowing peace of mind to pave the way for relief of her physical problems.

IS IT REALLY NECESSARY?

In recent years there has been a great hue and cry about "unnecessary" surgery of all kinds, from hernia repairs to heart operations, with hysterectomy having come under particular fire. Patients and doctors alike have criticized surgeons for being "knife-happy" and whipping out organs at the slightest provocation, for research, for practice, or (most often) for the money they will receive from the hapless patient or his insurance company.

Reputable surgeons disdain this hysteria as just the latest phase of the consumer complaint that has become almost a national pastime. But what is being done about it?

DOCUMENTATION For too long there has been little way for a doctor to prove that the hysterectomy *was* necessary when the patient claimed postoperatively that she had been operated upon merely for the surgeon's financial gain. Now, however, the establishment of Tumor Registries (offices in hospitals that keep records of all tumors removed and their malignant or benign states) has shown statistically that far more cancer has existed than was previously thought. Tissue from every operation is now examined microscopically, and every trace of cancer must be reported and recorded, so that the surgeon who indiscriminately cut out every suspicious uterus he encountered would quickly be discovered and dismissed.

PREVENTION Physicians and surgeons are watching each other as never before. All accredited hospitals are visited and inspected by officials of local health departments and by representatives of other hospitals. The American Medical Association has initiated the controversial "PSRO" (Professional Standards Review Organization), which provides constant checking for carelessness, unhygienic conditions, slipshod methods, and unethical practices. Some physicians chafe at having their shoulders constantly looked over, but PSRO is a fact of life and one that brings comfort to many patients who might otherwise question their doctors' propriety in taking to the operating room. And, of course, there is the constant threat of the malpractice suit, which can be brought by any patient against a doctor whom he believes has operated unnecessarily or prescribed unwisely. Malpractice insurance rates have soared, and the time and paper work involved in any suit make a physician more careful than ever to do only what is best for the patient in any given circumstances. The doctors are so careful, in fact, that the patient who is thinking of suing should think carefully *twice*—she is probably in the wrong.

SELF-PROTECTION The patient herself must be the final judge when it comes to selecting the physician and surgeon she feels will help her the most. If she has a trusted, long-time family physician, her trust is probably firm and unshakable. If she is consulting a specialist for the first time, she must do her best to follow the advice of physicians she already knows and trusts, and to use her own common sense. Is the doctor known in her community? What is his reputation? What are his credentials? What is the reputation of the hospital in which he operates? The answers to all these questions can be obtained from the local County Medical Society. The doctor's background can be looked up in The Directory of Medical Specialists, which can be found in any Public Library. And the patient is always free to "shop around" if she chooses, going from doctor to doctor until she finally settles upon one whom she trusts.

If she cares about herself and her family, she will be intelligently selective but not hypercritical, not using lack of a "good doctor" as just another excuse to side-step forbidding but necessary surgery. With checks and controls as strong as they now are, the patient seeking help has the best possible aids to selection of a physician, including the right to seek another opinion. She should keep in mind that the vast majority of doctors have their patients' welfare uppermost in mind—and her own welfare should be uppermost in hers as she finds a physician she can trust and then faithfully follows his advice.

CHAPTER 7

How Is It Done?

WHEN A WOMAN AND HER DOCTOR have decided to go ahead with a hysterectomy, a number of questions usually arise in her mind as to exactly what she's in for. If she has had previous surgery, she will be fairly familiar with the procedure and hospital routine, for hysterectomy is handled by the hospital staff in much the same way as is any other major operative undertaking. But for the woman who has never had an operation, or has never been hospitalized, the whole idea may seem grotesque and bizarre. Many people can take surgery in stride, but there are others who just plain hate hospitals and don't even like to visit sick friends. For the new patient, then, here are answers to some of the most frequently asked questions about hysterectomy in particular and surgery in general.

Who will perform the surgery?

Most gynecologists perform their own surgery, and the patient will know that she is being operated upon by a man or woman in whom she has already placed her confidence. If her doctor is not a surgeon, or if the problem is discovered and diagnosed by an internist or general practitioner, she will be referred to a surgeon, whom she will be able to get to know before the operation is performed. Of course, if she decides that she doesn't like or trust the suggested surgeon, she can always "shop around" and select another one. The patient is, after all, the "consumer" in such a situation. Although she should not postpone the operation indefinitely, or use dislike of a surgeon as an excuse to keep putting it off, she should be sure she has a doctor in whom she has complete confidence so she can go to surgery trusting that the best possible care will be taken of her.

Also present in the operating room during the surgery will be the anesthetist (whom the patient will have met and talked to previously), several surgical residents to serve as assistants, and operating-room nurses—not the same nurses who give bedside care, but specialists trained in surgical procedure and every facet of operating-room routine.

How soon before the operation must the patient enter the hospital?

This depends upon whether or not there will be any preliminary testing required because of the size of a tumor or because of any cardiac disease or other illness. If her general health is good, and if she has a normal, uncomplicated operation ahead, then the day before surgery should be sufficient.

What kinds of tests will be performed in the hospital before the surgery?

First of all, a complete blood count. Most people, whether or not they have had previous surgery, have had this test done at one time or another. Blood is drawn with a hypodermic syringe from a vein in the inside of the arm, and a tiny puncture is made in the tip of a finger, from which blood is smeared on a glass slide. From that point on, the patient has no more to do than wait while the technicians put her blood through a number of tests to determine her blood type, her bleeding time (how long it takes for the blood to coagulate), and whether or not she is anemic or has any other diseases of the blood.

A urine analysis, another familiar test, is also performed. As she does whenever she visits her gynecologist, the patient urinates into a cup or pitcher, and her urine is examined for sugar content (a high urinary sugar level is one of the first signs of diabetes), albumin (the presence of this protein may indicate a disease or may mean nothing), and any other signs of kidney disorder.

If the patient is more than thirty-five years old, an electrocardiogram will probably be ordered. Though many women will find this a new and strange experience, the test is neither complicated nor painful. Little metal plates, called leads, will be placed on the patient's chest, back, and arms and secured with adhesive tape over blobs of a clear gelatinous substance (called "electrocardiographic jelly," it looks and feels much like ordinary petroleum jelly). Wires go from the leads to the electrocardiograph machine, which records the actions of the patient's heart on a long tape. If she has never had one of these tests before, chances are pretty good that the reading will be completely normal. If there is any problem, though, now is the time to find it so that adequate precautions can be taken.

If he thinks it necessary to inspect the patient's kidneys, the physician may order an intravenous pyelogram. This, too, is a simple procedure. A nurse or technician will inject a contrast medium—a substance that shows up brightly on an X-ray picture—of the type that is very quickly absorbed into the urine. Then an X ray will be taken of the kidneys to determine whether the contrast medium flows through freely, as it should, or is somehow impeded.

Finally, especially in the case of a pelvic tumor, the patient may have to go through a barium enema test, a procedure that is not at all pleasant unless one happens to enjoy enemas. A suspension of barium (a contrast medium) is injected into the rectum and passes up into the intestines. Then an X ray is taken, and again the physician can follow the progress of the barium to see whether or not there is any intestinal blockage.

A chest X ray, of course, is routine and familiar.

Can the patient eat on the night before surgery?
Yes, she can have a normal dinner, but in most cases she will not be allowed to eat anything after midnight.

Will she be given sedation if she has trouble sleeping?
Absolutely.

When will the anesthetist visit her, and what will he say?
The anesthetist will pay the patient a call on the night before the surgery. He is not just a technician, but an M.D. whose specialty is keeping surgical patients unconscious and out of pain during operations. By examining the patient's chart and asking her about her history, he will be able to determine whether she has any respiratory problems or allergies that might interfere with the anesthesia. He will explain the procedure he has decided to use, and reassure the patient if she's nervous about it. Before he leaves, she will have to sign a form giving him permission to anesthetize her.

Must the patient sign any other releases before surgery?
Yes, she must also give the surgeon and the hospital her permission to perform the operation and to use their experi-

ence and judgment to handle any unexpected emergency that may arise. This is true of any operative procedure, and is done so there will be a legal, written record of the fact that the surgeon acted only with the patient's permission, or that of her husband or closest relative. Since a relative's permission is used only when the patient is underage or unconscious, or otherwise incapacitated, the hysterectomy patient can expect to do her own signing.

What will happen on the day of the operation?

When the patient wakes up, she may be hungry, but she will not be allowed to eat—this is seldom a problem, however, since elective surgery is scheduled for very early in the day. Either before she leaves her room or when she first arrives in the operating room, her abdomen and pubic area will be shaved by a nurse. This is done to ensure cleanliness, since bacteria can cling to even the tiniest hairs. Any woman who has given birth in a hospital or has had previous abdominal surgery will be familiar with this procedure, and yes, it itches when the hair is growing back—but not for long.

Either before or after the shaving, the patient will be transferred from her bed to a rolling table and strapped on as a safety measure. If she is apprehensive, she will be given a sedative at her request—many people ask for this and fall asleep on the way to the operating room, later remembering nothing. The table will be rolled to the operating room, where the patient will be eased onto the operating table. If she is still awake and aware at this point, the room and all its equipment may seem formidable, but she should know that everything she sees is there for her benefit. The large gas tanks contain oxygen and anesthesia, the straps and restraints are for safety's sake, to prevent her from falling, and the large lights that may seem blinding keep the operating field clearly lit for the surgeon and his assistants. The patient's abdomen will be painted, and repainted (although she probably won't be aware of it, having lapsed into unconsciousness) with an antiseptic fluid, and covered with sterile drapes before the incision is made.

The instruments come wrapped in packages that are sealed with striped tape—the stripes mean that they have been completely sterilized with steam. When the packages are placed in the sterilizer (called an autoclave), these tapes are plain—they have been specially treated so that the stripes will appear only when total sterilization has been achieved. There is no chance of unclean instruments being picked up by mistake.

All the stories about surgeons' scrubbing are true—after watching a scrub, one must wonder why their hands are not raw from the stiff brushes and harsh sterilizing chemicals. Their rubber gloves are also delivered in striped-taped packages from the autoclave, and the operators do not touch anything but instruments and the patient after they are gloved —if a glove happens to touch anything else, it is considered "contaminated" and is replaced. Absolutely every precaution known to man is taken to prevent infection and, these days, any kind of contamination in an operating room is very rare.

What kind of anesthesia is used, or does it differ? And how will it be administered?

It differs, and may be either spinal or general. If general anesthesia has been decided upon, it will be begun with sodium pentothal, the famous so-called "truth serum"—but no one need be afraid of revealing the family skeletons, for

in the dosage given for anesthesia it causes swift unconsciousness.

As the patient lies on the table in the operating room, one
of her arms will be strapped to a board that extends from the
table, and a needle will be inserted in the inner surface of
the arm, just below the elbow. A clear plastic tube leading
from the needle will be attached to a bottle suspended from
a rack above the table. As the bottle's fluid begins to flow
into her arm, she will quickly lose consciousness.

As soon as he is satisfied that his patient is unconscious,
the anesthetist will insert rubber tubes into her nose and
begin administering an inhalation anesthetic, or "gas." All
during the operation he will keep constant track of the flow
of the gas, the way the patient is breathing, and her blood
pressure. When the operation is over, the tubes will be removed and she will be allowed to regain consciousness.
Some patients find that their noses are stuffy for a few days
after this kind of anesthesia, but it is a minor irritant that
passes quickly.

If spinal anesthesia has been chosen, a needle will be inserted at the base of the patient's spine. The anesthesia will
be continually administered during the surgery, and the anesthetist will keep the same checks as during inhalation anesthesia.

*Is the hysterectomy performed through an abdominal inci-
sion or through the vagina?*

That depends upon the nature of the illness for which the
operation is being done. In most cases, it is carried out
through an incision in the lower abdomen, especially if
there is a malignancy or a tumor that is too large to allow
entrance through the vagina. Sometimes, when the vagina is

small or has been blocked, the surgeon will not have adequate room to remove the uterus through the vaginal route. Generally speaking, the vaginal procedure is reserved for those patients who also have to have an associated vaginal repair.

How long will the operation take?

That, of course, depends upon the nature of the problem and what the surgeon discovers once he has opened the abdomen. But an average, uncomplicated hysterectomy usually takes anywhere from fifty minutes to three hours, depending upon how much has to be removed.

How long should the patient expect to remain unconscious after the operation?

In most cases, she will not awaken until about an hour or so after she has left the operating room.

Where will she be when she wakes up?

She will probably say the classic, "Where am I?" because she will not recognize her surroundings. After the surgery has been completed, the patient will be taken to a recovery room, where there will be equipment to handle any kind of postoperative emergency, and where nurses are continually on duty. The nurses will administer oxygen and make sure that intravenous fluids are flowing properly. These fluids, glucose and water for nourishment, will be flowing into the arm through another intravenous tube—yes, there are a lot of needles involved, but they don't hurt after they're in. The nurses will also make the patient as comfortable as possible and make sure that she is breathing properly at all times. She will probably be pretty groggy at this point, and probably will not remember much about the recovery room.

How long will she remain in the recovery room?

If all goes well, her stay in the recovery room will not last more than a couple of hours—or until she is sufficiently awake and responsive to be returned to her room.

What are the aftereffects of the anesthesia?

Some patients may notice a feeling of nausea, and occasionally some vomiting may occur. Because muscle relaxants are used during the anesthesia, muscles sometimes ache a bit. In addition, there may be evidence of a condition called "atelectasis," in which some of the air spaces in the lungs collapse and need to be re-expanded. For this purpose, many patients are given "blow-bottles," into which they can exhale sharply—as in blowing up a balloon—to bring the lungs back to their preanesthesia capacity.

How soon after the operation will she see her doctor?

If there are no complications—and there seldom are—the doctor will pay his first postoperative visit at the end of the day or on the day after the operation. This depends, too, on his schedule and the patient's need for him to return.

How soon will she be able to eat and get out of bed?

Her first meal will be permitted on the second or third day after surgery, when she passes gas rectally, and she will probably welcome even traditional hospital fare by then. She will not lack for nourishment before that, though, since it will be provided intravenously.

She will be gotten out of bed—perhaps over her own objections—on the first day after the operation. Many patients complain about this, feeling that they need a few days to just lie on their backs and relax, but doctors realize that early exercise is important. The body is a hardy machine—

not only can it take early exercise after surgery, it needs it.
Exercise stimulates the circulation and is begun soon after
surgery to prevent any possibility of embolism (clotting)
and ensure the smooth and healthy flow of blood through all
the body's tissues. This early exercise will hardly be strenuous, however, and may consist of no more than walking a
few steps with a nurse's support.

How soon will she be able to have visitors?
In most cases, visitors will be allowed after the first postoperative day—but flowers and notes of cheer are happily
delivered any time.

*What about the scar? How big will it be, and how badly
will it show?*
The scar may be either horizontal or vertical, and will be
below the umbilicus or navel. Usually it is from six to eight
inches long, and will be a thin white line when healed, no
more or less visible than the scar from any other abdominal
surgical procedure. If the patient insists on wearing bikinis,
it will show; otherwise she need not even think about it.
Such scars are far less noticeable than the striae, or stretch
marks, that many women carry as permanent souvenirs of
pregnancy.

*How soon will the stitches be removed? Will this be pain-
ful?*
Some stitches, notably those used to close layers of skin
within the abdomen, are never removed at all but are so
treated that they are absorbed by the body during the
healing process; such sutures are called "chromic" sutures.
Nonabsorbable sutures used to close the abdominal incision
will be removed while the patient is still in the hospital, usu-

ally on the fifth to seventh day after the surgery. This is done quickly, and may tweak a bit—somewhat like plucking eyebrows—but is not really painful.

How much postoperative pain is there likely to be?

There is always a moderate amount of pain on the first night, but adequate sedation and pain-killing medication are always ordered. On the third or fourth day after the operation, some gas pains may develop as the stomach gets used to digesting food again. After that the pain usually subsides, although the stitches may be a bit sore for a while, or the incision may ache slightly. But as long as the patient remains in the hospital, relief will be available to her. After she goes home, her doctor will provide her with a prescription for whatever he thinks is necessary in her case.

How long will she have to stay in the hospital?

Generally, for seven to ten days if there are no complications. Most patients' chief complaint during this time is of boredom, and they are anxious to get back into action by the time they're allowed to go home.

Are there any special or unusual postoperative procedures connected with this operation?

Yes, another barium enema or a laxative may be given on the third or fourth day after surgery, to be sure the operation has not caused any intestinal blockage. Some patients find that they are not able to urinate for a short time after surgery, and if this is the case a catheter, or slim rubber tube, is inserted into the bladder through the urethra (the channel through which the urine normally flows). The insertion is sometimes moderately uncomfortable, but once the catheter is in it can hardly be felt unless the patient moves about a lot—which she is not likely to do at this point. Otherwise, there is nothing out of the ordinary as long as there are no complications.

What happens to the cavity in the body after the removal of the uterus? Do other organs move in to fill it?

First of all, the cavity to be filled is very small, indeed (remember that the uterus is only about three inches in length), unless fibroids or other types of growth have enlarged it considerably. In any case, segments of the intestines will naturally slip into the space left, so that there will be no "cavity" at all. The abdomen will very quickly resume a normal contour, which is, in many cases, a vast improvement over its preoperative shape.

Does ovulation continue after the uterus is removed? If so, what happens to the ovum—where does it go?

Whenever one or both ovaries have been left in the body, ovulation will continue, just as before. The ovum, however, having no uterus to which to travel, will simply disintegrate. With or without hysterectomy, this little egg is microscopic —only one cell in size—and it will just disappear as every unfertilized ovum normally does in the healthy uterus.

What should she do in terms of activity after she goes home?

Most patients are permitted to resume moderate activity within the first three weeks after they're home. A lot will depend on how she feels—but she should neither baby herself by becoming a self-imposed invalid nor push herself by engaging in strenuous activity too soon.

How long will it be before her activity can be returned to normal?

In most cases, patients can gradually work back to normal activity in about six weeks.

How soon can she go back to work?

Generally speaking, a patient can return to a physically sedentary job in about six to eight weeks; of course, if she's a teacher or nurse or holds some other kind of job that keeps her on her feet most of the time, it may be a bit longer before she'll feel like returning to full-time work.

How soon can the patient resume sexual intercourse, and is she likely to feel any difference or experience any difficulty?

Unless there are unusual complications, sexual activity can—and should—be resumed after six weeks. There is no physical reason for any change in feelings or sensations, nor is there likely to be any difficulty—many women even feel much better, knowing that unwanted pregnancy is impossible.

All of this information is based on the presumption that the operation is uncomplicated, of course, and since every patient is unique, each will have her own distinctive experiences. But, in general, this is an outline of what a woman can expect when she knows she has to have a hysterectomy.

CHAPTER 8

Bitter and Bright:
How Two Women Feel About Their
Hysterectomies

A HYSTERECTOMY CAN BE, but need not be, a traumatic experience that tears a woman's world apart and leaves her feeling depressed and lost. It should not be.

In the best of experiences, the operation means the relief of troublesome, if not downright gruesome, symptoms of some disease—often it is a rescue from a killer such as cancer. In the worst circumstances it is the natural response to an alarm that later turns out to have been false—a case of plenty of smoke where there wasn't much fire. In any case, it is—as is any major operation—an unexpected physical surprise for which the body is not prepared. Nature, after all, never intended for us to be cut open—surgery is the invention of man. But so is neurosis.

Animals cope instinctively with physical incapacity—they lick their own wounds, heal themselves, learn to walk on three legs instead of four. As far as we know, their emotions are immune. Animals simply adjust.

Humans, however, with all their intelligence—and its

stepchild, emotion—seem able to cope with physical trauma in widely varying degrees. The blind learn to read Braille, the paraplegic learns to use artificial limbs, the cardiac patient has begun to cope with artificial valves or even with another person's heart.

What, then, is so earth-shaking about the loss of a woman's uterus? Theoretically, nothing. Yet this operation more than any other (with the possible exception of mastectomy —removal of a breast) seems fraught with psychological stress. Women can lose an arm, a leg, a kidney, or a lung with considerably more aplomb than they can summon to deal with the surgical removal of a diseased uterus.

There is a unique psychological significance to many women in the loss of the life-giving organ. Many of them regard the uterus almost as superstitiously as did our ancestors, endowing it with the power to determine their femininity and identities as women. Others, more realistically and with far less emotional upheaval, can disregard its loss, considering themselves well rid of a source of trouble or potential death. As illustration, here are the true case histories of two women—one who deeply resented the operation and allowed it to make her miserable, while the other was glad it had taken place.

DIANE—"SHIRLEY TEMPLE TO HELEN HAYES"

The reaction of any given woman to an operation of this sort depends almost entirely upon her attitudes about herself and her life under external circumstances—those that have nothing to do with the surgery. This has become more apparent since the advent of legal abortion. Many women think no more of having an abortion than they would of having a tooth pulled or a wart removed; once it's gone, they forget about it. Others are haunted forever by guilt and thoughts of destroyed life; twelve years after the abortion they will look at every twelve-year-old they see and wonder, "What would my child be like now if I had let it live?"

So it is with the hysterectomy. While most women see it as the removal of a real or potential danger to life, others regard it as a loss of femininity. To them the female reproductive organs represent the essence of womanhood; once those organs are gone, so is the female identity. Such feelings of inadequacy can lead to identity crises that are never resolved—probably extensions of subconscious doubts that existed without the patients' knowledge. Fortunately, women with problems that intense can usually benefit from psychiatric care.

Other women, like Diane, go through temporary crises that they are eventually able to overcome without outside help. Such women are also the subjects of inner disturbances, but they possess a basic self-confidence that enables them to deal with their emotional conflicts logically and, in the long run, come out on top. Though they are in the minority, there are women who react to hysterectomy as did Diane:

At the time of her operation, Diane was forty-three. She had been divorced for ten years and had three children, aged seventeen, sixteen, and fourteen; all had been delivered by Cesarean section. A year after the birth of her youngest child, Diane had undergone a tubal ligation (tying off of the Fallopian tubes) for voluntary sterilization. Since her divorce, she has been working as a medical records librarian, a position that has given her access to an unusual amount of medical information, though she does not have a sufficient amount of education with which to interpret all of it accurately. Here, in her own words, is Diane's story:

"The reason for the hysterectomy came right out of the blue. I went to my internist for a perfectly routine checkup, feeling perfectly well, no symptoms of any kind. I had Pap smears and breast checks as always, and then the doctor did a perfectly routine pelvic examination. Except this time he detected what he said was a large growth. It was very big— later it turned out to be 5-cm. [about two inches] long. He said to me, 'The position of it is such that I can't tell whether it's an ovarian cyst or a fibroid—and this isn't my department anyway. I think you'd better see a gynecologist.'

"Now, this doctor is ordinarily a terribly self-assured sort of man, very calm. But suddenly he was really pushing me, and that scared me because I had been feeling fine and had no symptoms of anything. My doctor's getting so excited really disturbed me. Also, it had only been six months since my previous examination—I had had them regularly ever since I had had a D and C in 1968. And everything had been fine at my last examination.

"My doctor suggested that I see the gynecologist he usually recommends, but he turned out to be away on vacation. So he then suggested that I see Dr. S——, simply because he was in town.

"Dr. S—— made room for me very quickly, and I went to see him one very cold evening after work. He didn't know who I was, and I had only just heard his name because the recommended gynecologist was away. It was a Monday night, and that weekend I had had a terrible flu—as sick as I ever remember being. I literally could not move off the bed, and I was vomiting and very ill. But by Monday I was pretty much okay—I had recovered, gone to work, and then gone to see Dr. S——.

"His opening words constituted an apology for not having had time to find out why I was there or what the situation was. I told him roughly that my doctor was worried about a lump, and he honestly couldn't tell whether it was a fibroid or an ovarian cyst.

"He then did a very rapid but very thorough examination, along with a Pap smear and an on-the-spot estrogen count. Then he came into the office to tell me that he was quite concerned about me. At that point, on the basis of that one examination, he thought that it was a cyst, and that if it wasn't already malignant, it was probably becoming so. He also thought that it was hemorrhaging internally and that this was what had caused the severity of my illness over the weekend. Then he said that he couldn't be sure about it because of the scar tissue that had been left in the area after my Cesarean sections.

"The cyst, or whatever it was, was located in the lower right segment of the uterus. Apparently they couldn't pinpoint the location, and it was somewhat confusing. I never did get a clear story about it because, since they couldn't tell what it was, it must have been in a very awkward position. And there was so much scar tissue in that area anyway, I don't know how they ever even found the lump.

"But Dr. S—— was even more frightening than my doctor had been, and he insisted that I act on it immediately. He said that there was no time to lose—especially if it had already become malignant. My immediate reaction was that, if it was already malignant, there was no point in questioning time lost—too much time had already been lost.

"I was very badly frightened, and I had some very serious

reservations about going through any kind of radical surgery. Had I had a choice, if the malignancy had checked out, I probably would have elected to have chemotherapy for whatever amount of time I figured I had left.

"The next morning I called my doctor and told him what Dr. S—— had said. He was a bit puzzled, since he had not gotten that response—he hadn't thought I was that far gone. He said he would call Dr. S—— to check it out.

"Meanwhile, I called a friend who had had some reparative surgery done by a surgeon in whom she had great faith. She had a lot of problems with a Cesarean section rather late in life. I called her just to talk with her about what her experience had been like. But she became very alarmed. She made an appointment for me for that very day to see Dr. K——, who was the man who eventually performed my surgery.

"Dr. K—— said the same thing my doctor and Dr. S—— had said—that he really couldn't tell whether it was an ovarian cyst or a fibroid. And he's a gynecological surgeon. Now, that's interesting, that three such distinguished men really couldn't tell the difference between a fibroid tumor and an ovarian cyst. But he did say, 'You're so upset now that I wouldn't operate on you anyway.' And that in itself was pretty frightening. My youngest daughter was then fourteen—she's the baby—and what terrified me was the contemplation that something really serious might have been wrong with me, long before my children were ready to make it on their own.

"Dr. K—— told me to go home and calm down—he even gave me some sedation—and he said that I should go through with it just to be certain. I was already sterile—and I was forty-three and had three children, so I wasn't worried about losing the ability to give birth. I was divorced, anyway, and had been sterile for thirteen years, so I was quite well adjusted to that aspect of it.

"Dr. K—— suggested a radical hysterectomy on the basis of my not needing the organs. He didn't really think there was a malignancy, and he felt that there weren't enough other symptoms to warrant such a radical diagnosis. And I was really feeling in good health. There were no other problems—my periods had always been normal and regular. There wasn't even any appearance of the onset of menopause—nothing at all out of the ordinary.

"We waited for three months. Dr. K—— wanted me to have at least one more period and see what would happen. Then he did another examination, at which it turned out that the lump had apparently not grown—but it was large. The second examination was done in February, and then he did another one after my next period. Even though the lump had not grown, it also had not diminished in size—it became pretty obvious that it wasn't going to go away. So Dr. K—— felt that we might as well clear it up.

"At the time there wasn't much discussion about anything except my anxiety over whether or not it was really cancer. It seems to me that I spent more time thinking about whether they'd tell me if I really had cancer than I did about practical matters—such as what would happen to the supporting wall in the abdomen once the uterus was gone. These were things I wish I had had the presence of mind to ask about—or that someone had thought to tell me about.

"I received sedation from my doctor and from Dr. K——, and I was counseled not to be so hysterical. I must say that Dr. K—— was somewhat reassuring about the extent of the problem. But he couldn't tell me that it wasn't a cyst—he couldn't even tell me that if it was a cyst, it was or wasn't malignant. But he did say that there was nothing wrong with my breasts, and the blood tests showed that everything was all clear in that area. So I began to calm down a little about it.

"Still, left to my own devices, I would never have elected to have it. They kept saying to me, 'If we get it now, it probably won't be malignant. It's probably still encapsulated.' So I had a feeling of having a gun in my ribs—and I've certainly had that feeling since. Nobody ever once said anything to me about the possibility of any adverse consequences to the operation. Maybe they just assumed that because I'm a medical records librarian I was more sophisticated about medical matters than the average woman. But there's an awful lot we don't know.

"It never crossed my mind that anything could go wrong afterward. It just seemed that eliminating a possible breeding ground for cancer made an awful lot of sense.

"I remember resenting the fact that my doctor said, 'Just think, you won't have to have menstrual periods any more,' and things like that, downgrading the seriousness of the whole procedure. My periods had never been a big bother in my life, had never substantially interfered with anything. I had never regarded such things as problems, never had most women's troubles. I had had easy pregnancies, aside from the Cesarean sections, but I had recovered from those quickly, and I had breast-fed the babies normally. Because I had never had any problems, I really resented their attitude of 'Don't you want to get rid of all this mess?' What mess?

"We went ahead with the operation as scheduled. I checked into the hospital on a Sunday, and the operation

was scheduled for Monday. I had had several operations before, and nothing unusual happened that night. The anesthesiologist came to talk to me as they always do about things
like my teeth—they want to know whether you have any
fillings, or bridges and dentures that will have to be taken
out. I always have found the anesthesiologist very comfort-
ing—they come in and tell you what's going to happen, and
they're usually very nice. And of course they prepped me—
shaved the pubic area and gave me an enema.

"I do remember that the resident came in that night to
work me up. He asked a lot of questions and gave me the
most difficult pelvic examination I have ever had in my life.
He said to me afterward, very sternly, 'Well, now I understand why Dr. S—— and Dr. K—— couldn't make a decision as to whether or not you have a cyst or a fibroid, because it's really impossible to tell.'

"They gave me sedation that night—I'm not an easy
sleeper, I don't get a great deal of sleep ever. I certainly was
frightened about the possibility of cancer, but the operation
itself didn't disturb my sleep. I know a lot about surgery,
and I've been through it a number of times, so it wasn't an
unfamiliar experience. The only thing that's ever bothered
me about surgery has been the anesthesia. They usually give
you something that knocks you out—I think it's sodium pentothal. And knowing that made me a little nervous. I really
hate anesthesia—it takes you such a long time to go down.
But, as it turned out, with the pentothal it was very fast, not
so bad.

"We had decided when I had signed all the releases that
they would take everything—it was going to be a radical.
Both ovaries—the tubes, of course, were already gone—the
uterus, the cervix, the whole works. They said there was no

point in leaving any soft tissue, which could later become cancerous. Dr. K—— said to me, 'You're forty-three now. Suppose I only do a partial hysterectomy, then something develops and we have to go back in a couple of years and do it again?' And that did make a certain amount of sense.

"I did know that it would mean instant menopause, but then, again, I was forty-three, and knew that it would have begun in a few years anyway. Everyone had said, 'You just take estrogen pills, and everything is very simple.' I have a feeling that it was all made much too casual. People seemed to want to make me think it was just like falling off a log. But I feel terribly about it now. I felt that I just couldn't afford to take the chance. Now, of course, looking back at it, if I hadn't been so frightened I would have said, 'Let's check into it again in six months, and we'll talk about it again.' But I wasn't at all prepared to make that decision at that time. I kept thinking, 'If the doctors are right, I could be dead in six months.'

"The next day I was supposed to go into surgery in the morning, but I didn't go up until 1 o'clock. They had an emergency and had to use the operating room for that. I remember lying in the hall for a long time, and we were lined up as if it were Grand Central Station. So there I was, lying around all day, anticipating what was going to happen to me. Of course, by that time I was so groggy and sleepy that I didn't really remember much detail. They had given me a shot of something, and I was pretty much out of it.

"Once they took me in the operating room and administered the pentothal, I was out right away. The only thing I remember is that I came to faster than I ever had before, and there was a nasopharynx tube still in my nose—the doctor was apologizing because he would have to remove it. He said, 'Bear with us,' and they pulled it out. I don't recall having any pain at that time—of course, I was still pretty foggy. I think I went out again then, because the next thing I recall is being in the recovery room, where I stayed for quite some time. I came to in a criblike bed with bars on the sides—that's standard, it's just to protect you from rolling over and falling out of bed while you're still under the influence of the anesthetic. Someone came in periodically to check on me. There was a packing left in, but no drainage that I know of. This is a pretty straightforward operation—they just take it all out and sew you up.

"The first thing I remember when I woke up is that I was very much shakier than I had thought I would be. I remember that a good friend came to see me, and she had to feed me because I couldn't hold a spoon. They let me eat that evening—they brought me something, but I couldn't sit up and I couldn't hold a spoon. The nurse was sort of impatient, and she seemed to think that I should be able to feed myself. But fortunately my friend was there. That's all I remember about that night—I just couldn't negotiate very well.

"The only other thing I remember that hadn't happened to me before was that I had absolutely no muscular control. I remember soaking that bed about three times, and I was very uncomfortable because I had no way of knowing that it was going to happen. The poor nurses were absolutely beside themselves.

"They gave me injections of Demerol to take care of the pain, and my feeling was that they were giving me too much. I remember protesting at one point when I was uncomfortable—I wanted to see the doctor to find out what it was. I thought maybe some stitches were pulling. But they kept offering me Demerol, and I thought it was too much. Then they gave me sleeping pills at night, which were optional. The doctor gave the order, and I could ask for them if I had trouble sleeping. I think I must have made a fairly good recovery because I had a lot of company, and after a while I felt marvelous. I felt very relieved that it was all over with.

"For the first twenty-four hours I was awfully sick, but I think that was just the usual business of the anesthesia and the physical violence done to your body by any surgery. For twenty-four hours I was in very bad shape, but Dr. K—— came and told me I was doing fine. The lump had been a 5-cm. fibroid, not malignant. There was nothing wrong with me, and I was in good shape. I remember afterward wondering why I had been so excited about his telling me the truth right away, because I felt so badly I really wouldn't have been in the right condition to have heard it. Suppose it had been something terrible! I certainly wouldn't have been ready for it at that point. But I was so relieved to hear that there was no evidence of cancer!

"I had to stay in the hospital for ten days after the surgery. The pain gradually subsided—it never was unendurable. They have Demerol ready, and, if you need it, they give it to you.

"They tried to get me out of bed right away—within twenty-four hours. That wasn't very hard to take—remember, I'm an old pro at surgery. This was my fifth major operation. If you don't have a disease behind the surgery, such as cancer or something else very crucial, the recovery period is pretty much the same for hysterectomy and Cesarean section—you have gas, you're uncomfortable, and the stitches occasionally pull.

"But emotionally, I was terribly upset. I had the feeling that I'd never have any kind of a normal sex life ever again, and that kind of craziness. I didn't mention it to the doctors, though. First of all, the surgeon was not a man I'd discuss such things as sex with, anyway. He isn't the kind of person I'd discuss much of anything with. He's an excellent surgeon, but he's very patronizing. He's a very fatherly figure, but not the kind you can really open up to on a person-to-person sort of basis.

"Most of what I got was, 'There, there, you'll be fine,' as if he were saying, 'Don't worry about it, little girl.' And that I resented very much. This went from bad to worse. When I first went for a postoperative examination, he was talking about giving me hormonal treatments so I wouldn't have menopausal symptoms. Within about a month he had me taking Premarin—maybe that was too soon.

"My doctor told me that, because the operation would bring on an instant menopause, I should be receiving estrogen replacement therapy. He told me to expect hot flashes and feelings of some discomfort. And, sure enough, they began to occur shortly after I got out of the hospital. In the beginning they were quite severe, and they were such an unusual feeling for me. And it became even harder for me to sleep.

"My doctor really didn't give me much advice—I think he thought I knew more about it than I actually did. About the medication he told me that it came in different dosages and that it usually took a long time to work out the proper amounts. We started on the highest dosage, and this was where we came into our problems. Six months after the operation, I was a good twenty pounds overweight. And I'm a person who has never gained weight easily; I've always been lean, always lost weight quickly after childbirth, never been a compulsive eater. But within weeks after the surgery, I had shot up about ten pounds. I was frantic, in addition to any anxiety I might have had about myself as a woman —I think that sort of thing always follows this type of operation.

"Everyone had told me that my body would retain fluid, but that's one thing—I've had that happen during pregnancy. This was awful—I was suddenly getting to look like a tub. When I went back to my doctor and complained, his comment was, 'You're eating too much.' At this point I put myself on a crash diet, which was ridiculous because I had an ulcer. My doctor said, 'You're going to kill yourself. Stop this nonsense, stop this radical dieting and eat decently. I don't want you aggravating that ulcer.' But never once did anyone stop and say, 'Look, you're getting an overdose of hormones.' I had to start playing with the Premarin myself, taking different dosages. I had to be my own gynecologist, and that I resented bitterly.

"There was absolutely not enough information about what happens after this kind of sudden menopause—I'm not even sure they have it for someone who's going through a normal menopause. I have a very close association with physicians, and I think these were very competent people. But I do think that they ought to tell us enough.

"I had trouble and more trouble with the hormones over the next year. Finally, I took myself off it entirely because I figured I would rather have hot flashes than the twenty pounds overweight. And I immediately slid back to my normal weight.

"I don't think my voice has deepened—I've always had a fairly deep voice. There certainly is more hair growth—at least facial hair—but not much else. There was an awful lot

of 'up-and-down' feeling—like adolescence all over again. I
didn't know who I was going to be when I got up in the
morning. Sometimes I was happy, sometimes I was sad.
There were peaks and valleys that made it a very curious
feeling. I said to somebody, 'I'm the only adolescent I know
who's going through the menopause.' And my juggling of
the doses of estrogen didn't help either—it only compounded the felony.

"I think the thing that interested me the most about myself was my sexual reaction. I've never had any sexual hang-
ups—I've enjoyed my sex life. I've never had the idea a lot
of women have that it's a put-down—you know how men
are, they often treat you like an object—but to me it's always been a mutually enjoyable activity.

"But after the operation, I really kind of flipped—I suddenly had this crazy business about feeling that I was just a
receptacle, and that there was nothing there. It was so
weird for me.

"I asked my doctor about this, because he's really a kind
guy, and he'd say, 'Diane, you're crazy!' He'd say, 'Can you
have orgasms?' and I'd say, 'Yes, of course, but . . .' and
he'd say, 'Well, then, what are you worrying about? There's
nothing the matter with you. It's all up here in your head.'

"And yet I had some sort of sudden feeling that the parts
were all gone. It was tied somehow to the cycle—it made
me think of the drawings I've seen of ovaries and breasts
and everything being tied to the central nervous system.
Suddenly I had this feeling of, 'It's all gone, all these parts
of me are gone!'

"It's really very irrational, and I can't explain it rationally.
I was seeing a man at the time, and things were fine, there
was no practical problem. It was just that I felt I was only

half myself, and that I wasn't bringing as much to the sex act as I used to. I wondered what the hell I thought I needed an old, beaten-up uterus for, or who was going to inherit it when I died, but the feeling of loss was very strong for a long time.

"I would say it's only been in the last year or so that I've begun to relax. I've started seeing another man, and I think that has something to do with it. I'm much more closely involved with him, and I don't think he knows anything about it—he didn't live through it with me. I haven't felt any need to tell him about it. If we ever decided to get married, I'd tell him only if I thought he wanted to have children. But I've been sterile for thirteen years anyway, and the initial trauma of not being able to have children any more was over a long time ago.

"At the time I was sterilized I had had three children in four years, and the loss of fertility wasn't exactly a shock; it was something of a relief at that point to be sterile. That's when my sex life really took off—I've really had a good time since then. Besides, the problem of not being able to have children any more just isn't serious at my age. Most of the men I've dated already have children of their own or don't want any at their age. So I've never felt there was any necessity to tell them about my hysterectomy. There's no reason for the subject to come up, or for me to feel self-conscious about it. It was just immediately afterward that I felt sort of uptight about it.

"I got over the bad feelings just by living through them. The reassurance that there was nothing physically wrong with me was a help. If I had suddenly become frigid, I think I would have consulted a psychiatrist. But one of the dubious advantages of having lived a long time is the knowledge that 'This, too, will pass.'

"In retrospect, I'm kind of uptight about it. If they had just said, 'You have a fibroid, and we think you ought to have it out,' I'd have said, 'Later.' As far as I was concerned, I would have tried to live with a fibroid for years—and, unless it was unsightly or made me ill, I don't think I would ever have suggested having it out. It was only the threat of cancer that made me go through with it.

"The thing I'm most regretful about is that no one warned me about the side effects I'm now having. I'm about to investigate that—the bladder wall is inflamed, and there's some problem with the rectal wall. I have to go see what it is. It's fairly serious, and probably is going to mean more surgery. There's no pain, but there is an obstruction—I think it might be a hernia.

"I know that if anyone had warned me that this might happen, I would never have had it, even though they thought it might be cancer—I would have demanded further tests. Every patient should know enough to question her doctor about these things. She should ask about the hormones.

"If the problem were presented to me now that I know more about it, I'd first ask about the anatomy—the bladder wall and rectal wall, and what can potentially happen. This is particularly important for someone my age who's had three children—that area has already been pretty well worked over. And then I'd want to know all about the business of estrogen replacement. I am told by lots of people whom I trust that this is a very touchy area. Lately I've been seeing Dr. K——, and he and Dr. B——, my internist, are very conservative—neither one wants to use anything on me. Dr. K—— is the one who initially gave me the Premarin, but he's come to think that I should no longer take it.

"I still have hot flashes, but nowhere near as frequently.

They always happen when I'm emotionally upset or under pressure. But they do happen at least once every twenty-four hours. They've diminished considerably, in both intensity and frequency. Of course, you have your own built-in thermostat—I'm cold when everyone else is warm and vice versa—but apparently that's part of the whole menopausal picture.

"I think I'd like to know more about the pharmacology of the estrogen replacement. I'd like to know more about what happens to your body while all this is going on. I would have liked to have had it spelled out for me before I went into the hospital—like to have had more options and choices, more information about the pros and cons of it.

"I think that the misdiagnosis was terribly frightening. It was so frightening that, coming as it did, I wasn't able to think rationally about it. I could have lived with a fibroid for as long as I'm going to live anyway. They told me nothing concrete about the problems I might encounter, and how to deal with them.

"There is nothing written about the menopause for the contemporary female. All we know are vague stories about hysterical mothers and grandmothers, but there is nothing for the woman who intends to go on living a full life after the menopause—living and dating and continuing her sexual life. There's the picture of the crazy lady, or the involutional melancholiac, and I know I'm not going to be that. But I don't think anyone prepares you, tells you that it is going to be like adolescence all over again. One day you're Shirley Temple, and the next you're Helen Hayes.

"I wish that male doctors had a different picture of women. I don't think that contemporary females, with all our other liberation, view menopause the same way our grandmothers did, but nobody's written anything sensible about the fact that it still presents you with very real problems—sexually and emotionally. Your identity as a woman undergoes a great big change. If you go to a male doctor with menopausal problems, they just think you're crazy.

"As to cost, the hysterectomy itself cost about $450 in a New York City hospital, plus another $100 for the anesthesia.* The hospitalization was covered by my Blue Cross, but it must have run into the thousands for ten days. And I was approximately a month away from work.

"For a fairly young woman, it's a great shock to be suddenly plunged into middle age, and I think someone should prepare you for it. As far as the first frightening experience is concerned, I'm quite sure that the doctors meant well. But they just sat me down and said they thought I had cancer, and that scared the hell out of me. They should have said that they were concerned and then consulted my own doctor and let him tell me—someone who knew me. I couldn't tell my children that they thought I had cancer until after the operation and ordeal were all over with—I just explained that they had said I had a growth and had to have it out so it wouldn't turn into cancer.

"Not only did the doctors give me no counseling to help me get through it, but I've been under the impression—though that will always vary from person to person—that they're just not helpful about it. If anything, they're a little impatient about it. With a doctor, if something goes wrong medically, he's terribly concerned. But if everything is clean

* Costs, unfortunately, have risen since Diane's operation. A hysterectomy in a New York hospital now costs between $850 and $1200, and anesthesia about $250.

medically, he's not particularly concerned with your emotional problems."

Unfortunately, Diane overreacted to her experience in an emotionally damaging way. The way people respond to stress situations such as this is dependent upon each patient's individual makeup and upon her past experiences. Obviously, having gone through three Cesarean sections and one D and C, Diane was not really amenable to the idea of another bout with major surgery.

Note that she uses the term "radical hysterectomy" more than once. This is not only incorrect terminology, but rather extreme and inflammatory language. A true "radical" hysterectomy (also called Wertheim's operation) includes removal of much of the tissue surrounding the uterus, as well as part of the vagina. "Total" hysterectomy is removal of the cervix and uterus, whereas the excision of the Fallopian tubes and ovaries is a "salpingo-oophorectomy."

Diane's story does not make it clear just why her doctors insisted upon removing both ovaries. Presumably, they were afraid of leaving behind a "breeding ground" for future cancerous growth and believed that Diane was close enough to natural menopause that preserving a few more years of ovarian function was not worth the risk. In her case, however—and it has been pointed out that the surgeon was not familiar with her emotional makeup—it would probably have been much better to have left one ovary in and allowed her to go through a normal menopause in the coming years.

Diane was perplexed and shaken that "three such distinguished men really couldn't tell the difference between a fibroid and an ovarian cyst." However, it is a medical fact that no amount of reputation or experience can enable a gynecologist to make that distinction in a case such as hers.

As noted in the chapter on fibroid tumors, the fibroid can grow within the uterine cavity or outside the uterus. When it is inside, it can often be detected by palpation, and the diagnosis can be confirmed or refuted by dilation and curettage.

However, when pelvic examination discloses the presence of a lump outside the uterus, there is no nonsurgical way of determining whether it is cancer or not. Chances are good that it is, and to assume that it is a harmless fibroid and leave it alone is to gamble with the patient's very life.

The problem was compounded in Diane's case because of her previous surgery. As she herself said, "that area had been pretty well worked over." The lump could very well have been scar tissue that had built up after one of her Cesareans, or it could even have been a displaced loop of bowel. All the examining physician could tell was that there was a space-occupying mass located beside the uterus—a mass that could have been the ovary, a fibroid, or a malignant cancerous growth that could have been fatal.

Diane's doctor was honest with her. He said, in effect, "You have something there that shouldn't be there. You are forty-three years of age, and you had a Cesarean section fourteen years ago. You didn't have a tumor then, but you might have one now. If it's an ovarian tumor, you can't temporize with it; if it's a fibroid, you may be able to. If you don't strike out, if it's a fibroid, you will probably be perfectly all right. But if you do strike out, if it's cancer of the ovary, you are one hundred percent dead. You can't tell, and you certainly can't take the chance."

Diane's occupation made her particularly sensitive to misinterpretation of what her doctors told her. As a medical records librarian, she undoubtedly had access to a great deal of information—case histories, records, medical textbooks—

but she was not a doctor, nurse, or medical student and was therefore not properly trained to absorb and correctly interpret whatever she may have read. It's quite possible that she may have read a great deal about fibroid tumors and, when her lump turned out to be one, assumed that her doctors should easily have been able to identify it.

Basically, the surgeon operates for one or both of two reasons: to prolong the patient's life expectancy, or to improve her state of well-being. In Diane's case, the former was definitely the reason. As Diane pointed out, "I could have lived with a fibroid for as long as I'm going to live anyway," but she was also quite correct in thinking, "If my doctor is right, I could be dead in six months."

She was not correct, however, in using the term "misdiagnosis." In her case, no positive diagnosis was possible until after the operation had been performed. Unfortunately, Diane seemed to believe that her doctors were either dishonest or incompetent. But the fact is that any doctor could be possibly right or possibly wrong in such a set of circumstances. As a noted gynecologist has pointed out, "If you make an extraordinary diagnosis in medicine, you make it maybe once in a thousand times—and no doctor can go out on a limb when the patient's life is at stake."

Diane claimed that she would never have elected to have the operation performed. Actually, in her case, it was not a matter of electing at all; she had a problem that required treatment, and the treatment had to be carried out in the only way possible under the circumstances. The doctor gives his patient his advice, and it is, of course, her privilege to choose to disregard it. But he will give her the very best advice he can. Obviously, Diane's doctors tried their best to do whatever was possible to help her. It is unfortunate that she allowed herself to become frightened, but if she had had a malignant tumor, that very fear could have saved her life.

As to having "a gun in my ribs," another unfortunate choice of words that reveals the patient's panic, that is a matter of interpretation. How a given patient reacts will depend not only on the doctor's approach and verbal dexterity, but also on the patient's predetermined attitude. Eventually, it turned out that Diane had a 5-centimeter fibroid tumor—most probably one that had been growing for the last fourteen years. Because it was impossible to tell whether it was an ovarian tumor or a fibroid, hysterectomy was the accepted and justifiable procedure. Unless the doctor is absolutely certain that it's a fibroid—which would have meant following it along for quite a long time, with the attendant risk—a mass of that size does indicate a clear and present danger. In Diane's case—in which the mass just happened to have been found during a routine examination —it really wasn't safe to take chances.

Emotionally, Diane was very upset about her sex life at first. This is really very sad, since the actual sensations of the sex act have nothing to do with whether or not the woman has a uterus and ovaries; the erotic zones are entirely separate anatomically—and are also very dependent upon the emotions. There is an old-fashioned European idea that, if the cervix is left in, sexual expressions and feelings will be enhanced. This has never been proved, and is generally disregarded these days as being nothing more than superstition. More important, the cervix is often the site of malignancy, and if it is left in, there is always the chance that another operation may be necessary later to remove it—and it has nothing at all to do with sexual pleasure.

Diane did have a definite problem with her "instant menopause." Only her doctor knows why, with a patient of her age, he made the decision to remove both ovaries. Some doctors take everything out just as a matter of course, but for a premenopausal woman they could have left one ovary intact so that she would not have had to go through the sudden jolt that she did. She would, however, have had to go through a natural menopause in another few years anyway, and most women are able to accept that. They have known all their lives that it's going to happen eventually, and by the age of forty-three should be able to accept it as an inevitable and natural part of life.

It's quite possible that many of Diane's bad feelings and reactions may have had something to do with a feeling of sexual inadequacy that was there all along but was hidden and only brought out by the emotional aspects of her surgery. The majority of women manage to go through hysterectomy with no sexual problems. Diane's sex life, after all, is still a bit unusual for a woman of her age, notwithstanding the current wave of sexual frankness and freedom. Most women, by the time they're forty-three, have been settled down with one man for some time, or have resigned themselves to living without one. But Diane, as a divorcee, is still going through the courtship routine, meeting new men, leading the social and sexual life of a single, and available, younger person. This could easily contribute to a feeling of sexual inadequacy and even anxiety. When it is complicated by the loss of the female organs, it could be what brought about her feeling of being "just a receptacle."

Fortunately, Diane was able to get over bad feelings, as people usually do manage to survive traumatic experiences. Most of us learn to develop the necessary resiliency for coping with life's inevitabilities sooner or later. She noted that the men in her life had no complaints—those she's known recently don't even know about her hysterectomy, and she feels no need to tell them. Indeed, there is no reason she should.

When there is an emotional disturbance connected with a hysterectomy, it is often possible to correct it with the help of effective hormones. But every human being is an individual and will react in an individual manner to any type of medication. If this were not so, medicine would quickly be able to come up with a universal panacea for all of our ills— maybe even the common cold! Diane's doctors really had no choice but to try different dosages and see how her body reacted to them. They probably did exactly what they would have done in later years to treat her natural menopause.

A great deal of unhappiness is caused by the fact that so many people have received and propagated so much misinformation about the menopause, in both its natural and surgical forms. Many women dread its onset because they have observed or known about postmenopausal relatives or friends who have allowed themselves to become fat, lazy, and sloppy. Wrongly, these undesirable characteristics have been attributed to the menopause when, in fact, they are simply the result of a woman's having "let herself go." In Diane's case, her weight gain was simply—as her doctor told her—a matter of overeating, which could have been a result of her emotional distress. She probably didn't even notice that she was eating more than usual. But the hormones given to treat the menopause have no direct physical effect on body weight—again, there's the problem of misinformation. If a woman *expects* to gain weight after her menopause, she probably will.

The fact that Diane has nothing positive at all to say about her experience indicates that she went into it with the idea that she was going to suffer side effects. In truth, most hysterectomy patients just think of it as going into the hospital for removal of a tumor that could be malignant, and they're glad to have it out and harmless. But, in Diane's case, the operation seems to have brought about a feeling of castration, probably attributable to her way of life. It's never easy, after all, for a woman to bring up her children alone, and she is doubtless under a great deal of pressure, especially now that they're teen-agers.

It is understandable that Diane would be very anxious before the operation, knowing that the tumor might be malignant and wondering what would happen to her children if it should be fatal. The surgery was a gamble she had to take. Once it was over and she knew that she had been the victim of a false alarm, she apparently felt a letdown, a resentment that "it didn't have to be done after all," rather than the relief that would have come with the knowledge that it *had* been malignant and caught in time. But it did have to be done in order for her doctors to find out what was there. Undoubtedly she would have been much more anxious and upset walking around knowing that she might be carrying an active, cancerous tumor.

The operation was the lesser of two evils, but the greatest evil of all—the growth—was *there*. It could not be ignored. Leaving it in could have meant death. Taking it out meant the inconvenience, expense, and emotional turmoil of surgery and the loss of the organs, but the evil and its dangerous implications were gone.

It must be emphasized that Diane had had no symptoms

before her doctor found the lump. Had she experienced pain, excessive bleeding, or an unpleasant discharge, she might have been more grateful for the relief of her problems than upset over the method of relief.

A great deal of consideration is given to any woman who sees a doctor about this type of problem. But even when the examination is done with the patient under an anesthetic, only about 80 per cent of nonsurgical diagnoses can be accurate—and these are done by careful, experienced physicians. This leaves us with approximately a 20 per cent latitude of failure, even under the best of circumstances. It is obvious that no doctor can be as accurate as could be desired—no one can always tell beyond the shadow of a doubt. The situation has been likened to a far more common ailment, appendicitis: The patient with all the symptoms may *not* have an acute appendicitis, but then again he *may*. If he does have it, it's a fairly lethal situation. If he doesn't have it, he may be angered at having to go through an unnecessary operation, but it's a chance he's had to take in view of the strong possibility of real danger. All people, even doctors, occasionally make mistakes. And unfortunately, there just isn't enough time for the busy gynecologist to sit down and explain every aspect of every problem to every patient.

Diane is certainly correct, however, in her desire to know as much as possible in terms she can understand and interpret correctly. And that's what this book is all about.

To some patients, like Diane, hysterectomy is Trauma and Grief with a capital T and G, largely because of their own attitudes and methods of coping with life's unexpected obstacles. Others, like the woman next described, manage to maintain their emotional equilibrium, and even find ways to look on the bright side of adversity.

LEE—"TEN YEARS YOUNGER"

Lee had been a career woman most of her life—she was forty-two when she married Paul, a widower who had two children. Lee had always loved children but felt that, at forty-two, she was too old to bring new babies into the world. She said:

"When we were girls—my generation—nobody told us anything. Now people do tell young girls about sex. But I'm part of the generation that's helping the younger generation to catch up. Our mothers and other older people just aren't used to thinking about things like that—they shy away from it. But I think it should be told—every girl should know about the menopause and about hysterectomy.

"My feeling is that it's a very painful experience—a hard experience to get over. It takes a long time to get back on your feet again. I was extremely happy to have it all over and done with. And since I've been feeling well again—about the last nine months—I've been exceedingly happy and much freer. It was definitely, in my case, the right thing to do.

"I had had some troubles off and on. Paul and I have only been married for six years, and I was forty-two at the time of the wedding—still young enough to become pregnant by accident. So I thought it would be kind of interesting to take the birth-control pills. It seemed sort of a glamorous thing, this pill. I started taking them, but they didn't work for me.

"I took the pills because I didn't want any children and I

didn't want to take any chances. I had always wanted children, all my life, but I figured we were too old. Paul had his children from his first marriage, and there was no reason to start, at that point in our lives, raising babies.

"The pill just threw me all off. The pills are dated in the packages, but I found that I couldn't go more than ten or twelve days before I'd start menstruating again. I never did finish one of the packages—I'd start bleeding while I was taking the pills. It was a very bad reaction, as I've heard some women do have, so I stopped taking them.

"I switched to other methods of birth control, but from then on it seemed as though my periods began to be very irregular. Then, toward the end of the year, right around the holidays, I began to have very bad trouble with long periods. I was working at a large hospital then, at which they had a health service for employees, so I went to the health service and asked them what they thought I should do. They gave me an appointment for a clinic visit.

"When I kept my clinic appointment I didn't have any pain, just an awful lot of flow and bother. There was a young doctor at the clinic. I suppose he was a resident or an intern. All I remember is that he had big old nasty sneakers on, and I didn't like that somehow. He treated me a bit like a charity patient. And he said right away that I had fibroids, and that I should have an exploratory operation—a D and C —and an X ray and, if they found anything, which he suspected they might, they would have to go ahead and operate. He offered to book me into a ward bed.

"The young doctor didn't say whether the operation would be a hysterectomy or just a removal of the fibroids— he just said they'd do a D and C and, if they found anything, they'd 'operate further.' It scared me out of my mind.

"I pondered on it for a while. I certainly didn't want to go

into a ward, and I was pretty scared. So I talked to one of
the nurses in the hospital, and she said, 'Why don't you go
to one of our good OB-GYN doctors on a private basis?
Then, if you do have to have an operation, you'll be booked
as the patient of that doctor, get all your Blue Cross benefits
and employee benefits, probably have a private room, and
be sure of getting expert care.'

"So I went to see a gynecologist named F——, who had a
private office in New York, and I told him my story. I also
told him how scared I was. Paul went to the doctor's office
with me—by that time I'd gotten up enough courage to tell
him what it was all about. Dr. F—— went over me thoroughly and said there was no need to be alarmed. He
wouldn't even start me on hormone treatment. He said,
'Maybe a few fibroids, but many times they disappear.'

"I didn't think much about it. I just figured that, in a
clinic situation, they just do the quickest, easiest thing to
correct the problem. They apparently hadn't known that I
was an employee, and it hadn't occurred to me to make that
clear. The doctor who saw me probably didn't know anything about me but my name. I relaxed a little after having
seen the private doctor, and things got a little better. In the
spring I changed jobs—went to work as a publicity gal for a
medical college. I love the work, but I think it's for younger
women now—I just couldn't take all the running around,
chasing down stories. It takes a great deal out of you, and
then some. Now I've slowed down a lot—just do some writ-
ing and things like managing the commencement.

"The job transition wasn't difficult except that, all during
this time, about every three days, I'd start menstruating for
about eight days—that is, there would only be about three
days between these eight-day periods.

"So I went to the health service at the new job, and it was funny because exactly the same thing happened. They sent me to what they call the health group—it's a little set of offices in the middle of the hospital, where you're seen by a doctor who doesn't have an outside office. I was assigned to this young guy, Dr. B——. He's about thirty-seven, I guess, and he is one hell of a nice guy—this time no big sneakers.

"But plain talk. And he was very kind and understanding when I told him what had happened at the other hospital. I don't think he was ever soft with me in any way, not mushy or flowery, but he made me see that it was stupid to neglect my problem. It wasn't worthwhile to go on suffering from it and not do something about it. Again, the same procedure was recommended—first the D and C, then, if there was any need, the operation. We talked it all over and decided when I would go in—and that I would have a private room. I brought Paul up to meet Dr. B—— because I wanted him to know whose hands I was in.

"I went into the hospital in the latter part of July. I went in on a Saturday and had the D and C on Monday morning. Over the weekend they did all kinds of tests—I had an electrocardiogram and a whole series of blood tests. This was a training hospital for the medical college, one of those places where they have a lot of young doctors, residents, and interns, working with the patients. They like to give these kids practice in interviewing and taking records. So, even if you've been through this umpty-ump times, they troop in, maybe three or four at a time, to ask questions and write on big charts and act important.

"But Dr. B—— told me not to be bothered by them—and that I certainly didn't have to have any more internal examinations. I could refuse that. The pelvics weren't painful, but you feel funny when four or five of these young guys come in and all start peering around and poking at you. So Dr. B—— said I could refuse—just tell them that he had said I needn't go through that over and over.

"Actually, it was a very pleasant couple of days. Paul brought a bottle of wine in and stayed with me most of the time. I had a television set and some books, and I was really quite comfortable.

"Monday was fine. The D and C went off very well—it didn't take long at all. I was able to go downstairs and have lunch with Paul, and everything was normal. I didn't feel any different at all—no postoperative pain—but I stayed in the hospital while the decision was being made as to whether or not I should have another operation.

"Dr. B—— came to see me twice a day. Tuesday, an attendant came in and told me my abdomen would have to be shaved some more. I said, 'Well, it looks like I'm in for it,' and he said, 'Yes, the operating room's reserved for tomorrow morning.'

"Dr. B—— had told me way beforehand that it would be a hysterectomy, not just removal of the fibroids, but, I was a little upset by that because I hadn't quite figured it would be that automatic. He came to see me Tuesday night, and I said, 'Well, it looks as though you're going ahead.' He said he had decided that they had to get in there and see what the situation was. 'I know the fibroids are there,' he said, 'and they have to go, but I don't know what else is there, and I have to find out. I can't do that without operating.'

"I said something on the order of, 'This is quite a surprise,' and he said, 'Lee, I thought we had agreed that this is what I would do.' It was, that was true, but the sudden immediacy of it gave me some second thoughts. Dr. B—— talked to Paul and me together and said that this was the way they figured it: If the patient is a young woman, say, less than forty-five years old, still in her childbearing years, there would be grave doubt as to whether or not they should go ahead and do this. If she is between forty-five and fifty, half the doctors say, 'Do it automatically,' whereas the other 50 per cent say, 'Maybe yes and maybe no.' Dr. B—— said, 'I belong to the 50 per cent who believe that, unless there's some particular feeling you have about not wanting to have it done, we should go ahead and do it. By doing it, we're preventing all possibility of any future trouble.'

"He did say that it wasn't absolutely necessary to have it done right away, but why not? After all, I was there, I had had all the necessary tests, I was several days rested and in good general health. It seemed silly to leave the hospital and then have to go back later—we might as well go ahead.

"I remember that I asked him not to tell my husband if he found anything malignant—Paul had lost his first wife to cancer, and I couldn't bear the thought of his having to go through all that again. But Dr. B—— urged me to think it over and reconsider—after all, he said, who in the world would want more to help if I was in serious trouble? Now I think he was probably right.

"After the operation, he told me that he had left the ovaries in because they were in very good condition. But he hadn't said anything about that beforehand—that is, whether he would take everything or leave the ovaries. He explained that he might have to take them but he just didn't know what he would have to do until he could see what was there. As it turned out, there was a small cyst on one of the ovaries, but it turned out to be benign. The other ovary was perfectly healthy, so he decided to leave them both in for the sake of my own comfort.

"Wednesday morning, I had the operation, and after that

it was pretty much murder for a long time. Immediately after the surgery, I felt awful, absolutely horrible. They couldn't understand it. They kept giving me pain killers, but the medication just didn't seem to do anything to the pain. I didn't eat for two days—because they wouldn't let me.

"I had a catheter—that's a rubber tube into the bladder—and Dr. B—— got very mad about that. He came charging in and said, 'You don't need this thing any more,' and took it out, which was good.

"I was on intravenous feeding for two days, which seemed like forever. But I was coming along very well until Sunday, when a streptococcal infection of the urinary tract developed. Dr. B—— said it was because the catheter had been left in for too long. But he also said that people should not stay in the hospital one minute longer than was absolutely necessary. He said, 'I send my patients home as soon as I possibly can because a hospital is a place for sick people, and if you stay here while you're getting well, you're liable to catch something.' He was most anxious to get me home, but with the infection my temperature went up to 104°, and I had to stay another couple of days. I really was in bad shape for a while there, and I had terrible pain.

"I stayed until the following Wednesday, and then Dr. B—— insisted that I go home, whether the infection was cleared up or not. And it wasn't, it was still terribly painful. It was quite an ordeal just getting dressed and getting out of there, but I went home, where I stayed on a couch for the next two weeks. I couldn't even get up to answer the telephone. Then I had a terrible reaction from the penicillin I was taking for the infection. I had never been allergic before, but suddenly I was—welts broke out all over my neck and back. Never again.

"When I went back for my checkup, about two weeks later, Dr. B—— said I seemed to be okay. Paul was most anxious to get me out to our farm in the country—he thought it would do me good. The weather was lovely by then, the beginning of autumn, so we took off as soon as Dr. B—— said I could travel. We have a little sports coupe that has leather bucket seats and is very comfortable to ride in— I don't think I could have stood the trip in a regular car. It was a long and trying trip, but we were glad to get out there.

"I stayed pretty quiet and inactive all the time we were out there—we stayed for four weeks, and Paul did all the marketing and cooking, bless his heart. He took such good care of me, but I had no strength—I don't know if it was the infection alone or the combination of that and the operation, but it certainly had me down.

"Emotionally, I felt okay. As a matter of fact, I didn't think much about it from that angle. Of course, I felt tremendous relief when Dr. B—— told me that he had found absolutely nothing wrong or malignant, and that I would never have any more trouble, never have to have another operation of this type. I think all women probably have some kind of fear of cancer. My grandmother was a Christian Science practitioner, and my mother was raised as a Christian Scientist, although later in life she got away from that kind of thing. But my grandmother died of uterine cancer because she wouldn't do anything about it, never would acknowledge the fact that there was something wrong with her. I think that's an extremely bad way to die. I know by the way my mother told me about it that it really must have been terrible.

"I think this is very important, because they take those things down when they take a case history, and some day they may find that there's a pattern to it—X number of cases in which the grandmother had cancer and it skipped her children and was passed on down to the grandchildren. Maybe I think about these things because I work in a medical college, where everyone is so aware of all the things that can happen to people. We're all bats about Pap tests—I used to have one regularly every six months.

"Everyone there is very conscientious about tests and checkups, and very conscious of all the illnesses that can beset us. So naturally it was a very great relief to know that nothing further could happen to me. I'm assured now that it can't.

"I didn't have any bad feelings about myself as a woman. But I did feel badly about myself as a person. They gave me a nice long stretch of time away from the office, a leave of absence, but soon the time came when I realized that I had to go back. I tried to go back as cheerfully as I could, but I still didn't feel well. I had an awful lot of trouble with the inner stitches. Every time one of those stitches broke loose, I'd have awful pain. One day it would be on one side, the next day on the other. Dr. B—— told me all I could do about it was lie in a hot tub and soak, but even that didn't do much good. I just had to go through it and wear it out.

"Getting back into the work routine and the atmosphere of the office was very difficult. Suddenly I was plunged into great activity on all sides, and I couldn't do it. I was just lost. I was like a mushroom plopped down in the middle of everything that was going on around me. I simply could not cope with it.

"Nobody expected me to cope with it at first, so I wondered why I was worrying about it. But after a couple of weeks I found myself back at the health group with Dr.

B——, weeping. He, as I said, is a very practical young guy, and he said, 'What are you crying for? Do you think you're sick? Do you think there's anything the matter with you?' I said, 'No, I know I'm all right, everything's okay, but I just don't feel like myself.'

Dr. B—— told me, 'Look, Lee, you can assault the human body just so far without the body rebelling against the assault. And that's what's happening to you now. We've really done a job here, and it's a good job, and we know it had to be done, but it's going to take your body a long time to adjust to it.' He gave me some pills, an estrogen, and said I probably should keep taking them for three or four years, maybe all my life. They're nothing, just little tiny pills.

"Fortunately, I didn't have any side effects. But Dr. B—— asked me about our marital relations, whether or not we had resumed. When I said yes, he replied, 'That's *very* good, and it's very important.' I found that very interesting—he told me that you start certain things going during intercourse that are very healing for a woman in this condition. He said, 'Don't hold back on any of that kind of action for fear that damage might occur, because love-making is extremely beneficial.' I thought that was really very nice to know.

"It's funny, my mother asked me whether the operation would prevent us from having marital relations, and I was appalled. That's what I mean about the older generation being ignorant. People should *know* these things. I've often thought since then that, if doctors had a little bit more sense, they'd know more about the way to talk to women about this sort of thing.

"For example, if they'd explain that the thing they're taking out is just a little, pear-shaped organ, I think the whole thing would take on more natural proportions in the patient's mind. In the same way your mouth magnifies things through taste, and your fingers magnify things through the sense of touch, a woman's mind magnifies the importance of that part of her body. Her mind is pervaded with the idea that something great is gone. But something great *isn't* gone. It's just a little, worn-out, organ that might just as well go.

"As Dr. B—— said to me, 'What do you need it for?' and, of course, he was right. Now that it's all over and I'm adjusted to it, I feel extremely happy about it.

"It's important, of course, that I wasn't concerned about wanting children. Even though I love children, and have a kind of longing in my heart to have something of mine around, it's too late now. If we had a child now, we'd be sixty-four by the time he or she was twenty—I just don't think that sort of thing is fair to the child. Besides, not everyone is cut out to cope with children, especially in their fifties. I adore my nieces and nephews, but I really don't like to have them around too terribly long. They kind of get on my nerves.

"There are many ways, I suppose, with which I have resolved the childlessness business in my own mind. Once you've settled that, for one reason or another, it's a great relief to have this operation over with.

"I finally had to come to grips with the problem about my work—I just wasn't producing what I was expected to do. I was just not able to function at the office. So I started working a three-day week—I worked Tuesday, Wednesday, and Thursday, so that Thursday night Paul and I could take off and go to the country and stay through Monday. Of course, I didn't get paid for more than three days a week, but I didn't mind—it gave me a sense of freedom.

"Fortunately, the operation had not been a financial burden to us. The hospital was paid for by Blue Cross, and the rest of my expenses were taken care of by my employee benefits. Dr. B——'s bill was taken care of by insurance—$750 for the operation. There was just the anesthetist's bill, the television set, and the telephone, and that was absolutely all. No problem.

"When I began working three days a week, my boss and I had a long conversation, during most of which I cried. But she was very understanding—she's about fifty-six herself, so she's been through the menopause and knows what a hard time it can be. The shock to your system and the absence of the monthly periods is a complete change. And something happens that I can't account for. I don't think anyone can quite explain it—it's a *mind* thing, very nebulous. But it's a feeling of inadequacy.

"So when I finally had this heart-to-heart talk with my boss, more like a sob-session, I told her I just couldn't go on. She told me there must be an answer to this someplace. She sent me to her doctor, an internist, very fine man—at that point I even had thought I might need a psychiatrist. But my boss said, 'If you do need a psychiatrist, this doctor will know it right away. You just go see him and tell him your story. But I think all you need is some more help. Maybe with that and the three-day work week, everything will be all right.' I thought that was extremely kind. I was very much touched by it.

"I did go to her doctor, and he was terribly nice. Again I went through all the history, and asked him if he would take me on, if I could count on him for just general purposes. I told him that I liked Dr. B—— very much. This doctor, Dr. E——, said that all I needed was a little help by way of a kind of 'tranquilizing pill with a little bit of a kick to it,' as he described it.

"He gave me the pills and told me to take one in the morning and one again in the afternoon if I needed it, and one at night if I needed it. I started taking them regularly in the morning, and one in the afternoon if I began to get nervous after lunch in the office. Pretty soon I began not to need the afternoon one, and, after about a month, had given them up altogether. It was really just what I had needed to coast me over.

"At the end of the year I decided I really liked the three-day work week, and Paul had retired from his formal business, so I decided to stay on that basis permanently. Now we've been having a really great year—going to the country every weekend, having ourselves a ball.

"At the time, it was a very bad physical experience, but in general I'm extremely happy about it, very glad we went through with it. I feel absolutely about ten years younger. I think it's very worthwhile, and if you're in the right hands, there couldn't be anything more beneficial. With all the circumstances that I've outlined, if you've made up your mind that you don't want any more children, and if you have faith in your doctor, nothing could be more satisfactory—and right. It relieves so many fears.

"I think it's very important to emphasize that sex is so very much better—much more comfortable, and much freer. I think this is partly Paul's feeling and partly mine—he feels that I'm well and good again, and he doesn't have to worry about me any more. The other freedom comes from my half of the contribution, and together they make it good. We've been very much in love for a long time, and we've been very good together—and recently I've been noticing that everything has been happening for us in a much more *fun* way. So much freer.

"Rather than ending my sex life, or feeling like an invalid or incompetent, I suddenly feel kind of young again—but without all the worries that you had when you were a kid."

Lee had a few bad moments and the pain that is inevitable with any kind of surgery, but she was able to overcome her difficulties and adjust quite well to being without her womb.

Her problem with birth-control pills was undoubtedly caused by the low dosage that was originally prescribed for her. About 20 per cent of all women react this way to the low-dosage pills, not being able to get through a cycle without beginning to menstruate. In most cases, the problem is remedied by simply increasing the dosage. But, in her case, she neglected to go back to the doctor who had prescribed the pills, and just stopped taking them. Her later menstrual problems were probably related to her fibroids.

When she decided to seek medical help, it was unfortunate that she chose to go to a clinic, where she was probably seen by a very young and inexperienced doctor. She resented being treated "like a charity patient," and was irritated by the doctor's "big old nasty sneakers." It is true that most clinics are staffed by beginners, and that many of the patients are, in fact, recipients of charity. The personnel apparently were not told that she was an employee of the hospital, and she was treated in the routine, assembly-line fashion that is standard practice in such places. Had she chosen to see a private gynecologist, which she certainly could have afforded, she would undoubtedly have received a much higher caliber of care.

In the long run, however, Lee came through her experience very well. She had a loving, sympathetic husband and a good understanding of herself and of the fact that her femininity was not contained in the "little, worn-out organ" that she lost to surgery. Because her ovaries were left intact, which they should be whenever possible, she does not experience any hormonal imbalance and will be able to go through a normal menopause, just as she would have if the hysterectomy had not been performed.

Despite the obvious differences in their experiences, Diane and Lee had two very important things in common: first, an initial and intense reaction of fear, and second, the belief that all patients should be told and made to understand more about the operation than they generally are.

The fear is natural and inevitable. Any person, man or woman, faced with the possibility of cancer, is going to feel the grip of fright with which we all have been conditioned to react to the idea of death. If there is anyone who is *not* afraid of cancer, he probably doesn't know what the word means.

The fear can be lifesaving, though, even while it is churning our stomachs and robbing us of sleep. Without it we would blithely expose ourselves to all kinds of risks, and the national life expectancy would be considerably lower than it is. With the fear, we *act*—not always wisely or rationally, but we are jolted out of lethargy by the most forceful protective mechanism we know: the will to survive.

Both Lee and Diane were scared "out of their minds." Both acted on their fears. Both are still alive.

Both are also correct in the belief that patients should be better informed, for nothing is so fearful as the unknown. Today physicians have, for the most part, discarded the aura of mystique that has for so long made medicine virtually synonymous with magic for many laymen. Few doctors will be unwilling to explain the basic whys and hows of a procedure to their patients, provided they are not bombarded with panicky and repetitive demands for minute details and promises of miraculous cure. Doctors know that a well-informed patient is likely to be more cooperative and thus derive greater benefit from whatever treatment is necessary. On the other hand, the patient who makes a pest of herself with endless and pointless queries will only succeed in hindering the physician's best efforts to help.

Any patient who faces possible surgery should be prepared to ask pertinent and intelligent questions, listen carefully to the answers, and accept reasonable explanations. Self-education is an excellent weapon against a fear that can be crippling if not conquered, and vast amounts of information are now available via books, magazine and newspaper articles, films, and television programs.

Even conversations with friends can be informative, although the prospective patient should be careful to shun old-wives' tales that can feed fear and produce grotesque misconceptions about the aftermath of hysterectomy. "My daughter-in-law grew a mustache" from a superstitious neighbor is no reason for the surgical candidate to contemplate buying a razor—if the daughter-in-law actually *did* grow a mustache, chances are good that her mother had one, too, and that the problem was hormonal and hereditary, not surgical.

Lee's comments about the generation gap are interesting in that most hysterectomy patients are older women—those whose mothers told them little and who may be subject to all kinds of superstitions and unfounded legends about hysterectomy. Hopefully, things have changed enough that patients of the next generation—or even the next few years—will be well-informed and equipped to take the operation much more easily in stride than their unfortunate mothers and grandmothers.

CHAPTER 9

Nature's Balance

IN AN EPISODE of the popular television program "Maude," the title character lay wide awake and tormented in her bed, listening to her husband snore peacefully and trying to decide how to break to him the news that she had to have a hysterectomy.

In a previous, highly controversial and widely publicized program, Maude, a mother and grandmother in her late forties, had elected to have a legal abortion rather than another child. The show prompted such a hue and cry of outraged morality that a number of local stations refused to show it, and the network was bombarded with mailed and telephoned complaints. Doubtless many viewers chose to believe that Maude's current predicament was a form of the divine retribution with which she frequently threatens her husband: "God will get you for what you're thinking, Walter."

Medically, of course, there is no basis for such a belief. Abortion, properly done, does *not* bring about the need for a hysterectomy. Maude, like most hysterectomy patients, had fibroids.

Most of the program consisted of Maude's blundering

efforts to speak the fearful words. Finally, after having revealed her "awful secret" to Walter, and having been reassured by him that her health was paramount and the operation would have no adverse effect on his feelings for her, or on their love life, Maude returned to bed. Instead of falling asleep, however, she continued to stare at the ceiling and eventually sighed, "Good Lord, we're going to have matching mustaches!"

The line drew a good laugh from the studio audience, but it's likely there were many home viewers on whom the humor was lost—women who still believe that hysterectomy is synonymous with masculinization or, at the very least, a diminution of femininity. By now it should be obvious that this is simply not true; that femininity comes from within each woman's mind and personality and cannot be squelched by the simple removal of a few diseased internal organs.

The durability of the feminine nature is well-known but depends, in each woman, upon the individual's belief in herself—not only as a woman, but as a person. In most, femininity is so deeply ingrained that it just "comes naturally." Unless a woman allows fear and self-doubt to erode the "self" in which she has spent her entire life, no dramatic changes will take place. In any case, no bulging muscles, swaggering gaits, or deep voices will develop as results of a hysterectomy. And no mustaches will grow.

Maude should have talked to Sylvia, a real-life woman who, in spite of her later dismissal of her own fear as "madness," did at one time harbor a horror of hairiness. Having overcome it, as well as other fairly typical problems associated with hysterectomy, Sylvia has emerged as an excellent example of a patient for whom the operation was a complete success and the spirit didn't die. Thirteen years after her hysterectomy, Sylvia is, in fact, so secure and well-adjusted that she asked that her real name be used, declining the offer of anonymity accepted by the other patients interviewed for this book.

Six months after her final gynecological operation (removal of the last remnants of her only remaining ovary), Sylvia is forty-four years old. Up close, she looks about ten years younger; from across a room, especially when, on casual occasions, she wears her hair in pigtails, she could pass for a woman in her twenties, an image that is enhanced by bright eyes and an infectious laugh. Not giddy or flighty, she nonetheless obviously derives the most out of life and enjoys herself tremendously.

Sylvia is no Pollyanna, one who could dismiss the entire business with an airy wave of an uncaring hand and pretend that nothing had ever happened. She went through what she calls "my own private little hells," and needed some help in coping with them. But she believes strongly that, for the most part, they need never occur for women who are better-informed and prepared than she was for the operation and its consequences.

For Sylvia, trouble began early when, at the age of eleven, two things happened almost simultaneously: She began to menstruate, and fibroid tumors were discovered. It was, as she puts it, "a terrible experience for a child." For the next eleven years she was in and out of hospitals, having tests and D and C's, until, when she was twenty-two, her left ovary was removed.

Fibroids are quite unusual in a child of eleven, and when they happened to Sylvia, more than thirty years ago, much less was known about them than is known now. Moreover, they were not something that could be discussed openly, particularly not with a child. As Lee pointed out in Chapter Eight, "People just didn't talk about such things in those days." Sylvia was left in the dark, knowing only that she was a very sick little girl.

"No one ever explained any of it to me," she says now. "I was just sort of slipped out of the house so the other children wouldn't know where I was going, taken off to a doctor, and left to handle it pretty much by myself. No one told a twelve- or thirteen-year-old child what anything was about—*no one.*"

In retrospect, however, she believes that her childhood experiences with illness and hospitals held advantages-in-disguise that, without her knowing it at the time, prepared her for the life she was to lead as an adult.

"Some children who have spent many years in hospitals become more creative or accomplished than the others," she asserts. "You are put aside, you are a special person. I think of myself now as having been exceedingly lucky to have had all those experiences. My sisters and brothers went to school at the usual times, while I was in the hospital getting the best of everything. I was encouraged to read, I was encouraged to use my mind rather than my physical being to do things. I was given all the advantages that a normal child wasn't, as far as being creative was concerned. The theater became very important to me and, through the theater, films."

By the time she was twenty-two and had to have the first ovary removed, Sylvia had begun her career in the film business, having abandoned a brief but less-than-enthusiastic attempt at working for the stock exchange. "Oddly enough," she recalls, "the operation sort of coincided with my decision to really try and make it in film production. I think I may have made up my mind subconsciously, even then, that I would not be having children."

For several years she worked in the animation field, "inking, mixing paints, doing what I was told, learning the business. Back then I was 'the kid,' the lowest face on the totem pole." The loss of the ovary was not particularly traumatic at that point—another operation, another hospitalization—and no need yet to face the possibility of being childless.

During the next few years, Sylvia married and, for a time, did try to have a child. She saw a number of doctors, had all the tests, and did have one pregnancy, though she lost the fetus in the second month by spontaneous (natural) abortion. Now she reflects, "I obviously was not meant to have children."

The spontaneous abortion did not throw her off balance as much as might have been expected. Guilt was not a factor since, after all, she had tried, and the failure had not been anyone's fault. At the time, she explains, "I pretended to be very upset and concerned, but the absolute truth was that it was something of a relief. I was so busy learning and doing that I did *not* want to take time out to have a child, knowing the ensuing years would be taken up with raising it."

Years later, when she and her husband broke up for reasons that have nothing to do with her gynecological problems, Sylvia saw it as a fortunate stroke of fate that there had been no children. "We would have split up anyway," she is sure, and "think what it would have been like to have been alone with a child and still trying to accomplish the things I was reaching for." Nature, she felt, had achieved a balance.

When she was thirty, however, Nature struck a blow that

settled the question once and for all. The fibroids had re-
curred to the extent that she had to undergo a hysterectomy,
removal of her entire uterus and most of her remaining
ovary, leaving just enough to provide the ovarian production
of hormones that would save her from having to go through,
at an early age, a premature menopause. But the finality of
it brought about an unexpected reaction.

Sylvia had no physical problems at all with her hysterectomy. But superstition got in her way in spite of herself.
Like Maude, she had visions of shaving cream.

"I think the importance of this book is to dispel the
bugaboos that every woman has," she says. "Every woman
I've ever talked to who's never had a hysterectomy has been
influenced by one, at least one, of those awful Old Wives'
Tales. Did I have any? I didn't think so at the time, but of
course I did, we all do. Mine was the mustache.

"I sort of wondered, offhand, if I might become a little
more hirsute. It wandered around in the back of my mind:
Will I get a mustache? Madness! Absolute madness that in
this day and age such a thing should even occur to me! I
never even asked my doctor about it—part of me *knew* it
was ridiculous, and that the doctor would probably have a
good laugh on me if I were silly enough to bring it up."

Of course, Sylvia did not grow a mustache. But another,
far more real fear did give her serious concern, as it does
any woman who is faced with a hysterectomy, regardless of
what her doctor may have told her. Asked whether she had
been afraid of the possibility of cancer, Sylvia replied:

"I think anybody who says 'no' to that question is a rotten
liar. Of course it enters your mind, even if the doctor has
told you it definitely isn't cancer. After the first operations, I
was horrified it was cancer, because they had gone in there
too many times.

"By then I was an adult, a lone, thinking adult, with no help from the outside, and the fear was churning around in there, driving me mad. Getting rid of it was a triumph for which I needed some help. Finally I realized that, if you *do* have cancer [she didn't], that's the least dangerous place to have it, because they can get rid of it all if they catch it in time. In any other part of the body, the liver, the lungs, the vital organs, you get cancer and that's *it*. But the uterus is definitely an expendable organ."

As she mentioned, Sylvia did need help. After her hysterectomy, she was plagued by a depression she was unable to explain to herself. She was happily married, she had no conscious desire for children, her career was blossoming, everything was going beautifully—and yet she was terribly depressed and didn't know why. Eventually, at the suggestion of her surgeon, Sylvia sought psychiatric help.

She went into therapy for a little less than a year, which is quite a short time as psychotherapy goes. Typically of one who works in a business such as films, she expresses her eventual realization of her problem in visual terms:

"The strange thing about an operation of this sort is that you can't see what you're missing. You can lose a hand, a toe, a foot, and you can *see* the result, you know what's been done. But when they chop something internally, there's no visual aid to convince you that it's done and over with. So mentally you can bury that in the back of your head and not know what's bothering you.

"As an illustration of what I mean, during that time my husband and I were on the road a lot, and for almost a year after the hysterectomy, without even realizing what I was doing, I was carrying a Kotex belt in my suitcase. One day my husband was unpacking for me, which he had never done before, and he found it and said, 'What the hell is this?' I said, 'It's a Kotex belt—gee, I don't know why I'm still carrying that thing around.'

"I think that points out very clearly the fact that something hidden was bothering me. It was not yet a reality to me that I could not have children, definitely not a reality. The incident sort of shocked me, and because of that and the depression I was going through, I went into therapy.

"It was not a prolonged therapy, and it was fairly easy once we found out what was buried. And that was, of course, the fact that I couldn't have children. But by that time in my career, I had advanced to the point at which I was saying, 'Thank God I don't have children. How could I have had children and do what I do?' I couldn't have. And I came to the realization, of course, that now I could throw the Kotex belt away. And I did. That helped.

"Even though I had not really wanted children, the fact that I *couldn't* have any was a knowledge I had just tucked away somewhere and left to fester until finally the therapy located it, brought it out. Then I was able to acknowledge what had been bothering me.

"Finally the 'limb' was gone—like an amputated foot, I could 'see' what was missing. Surprisingly, it came out of my own mouth—probably led by the doctor, but it was my own realization. Sure, when a limb is removed they say you can still feel it for a while, but your eyes are helping you to solve the problem. But in there, you don't know. You have *never* seen it. You haven't seen that uterus ever in your whole life, so how can somebody tell you it's gone? It's something that I think women have to wrestle with all by themselves if they don't get some sort of guidance."

Fortunately, the guidance that Sylvia sought did the trick for her, as it has for so many other women. After less than a year of therapy, she had resolved her regrets and feelings of loss and plunged back into her film work.

"Is my life a good life?" she muses now. "Well, it's good for *me*. And it works for me. And the events that have led up to this and the events that have occurred since the main operation seem all a part of the pattern. It worked out beautifully for me—and that's really what it's all about, isn't it?"

After her hysterectomy, another thirteen years went by before Sylvia had to begin taking estrogen replacement therapy. During that time she became very successful in her career and advanced to the position of director/producer for the documentary film company for which she works. She also re-entered the world of singles, having ended her marriage for personal reasons that, she emphasizes, had nothing to do with her hysterectomy. As a single woman, she found that her operation made no difference at all in her subsequent relationships with men.

"No man in my life has ever reacted badly to the knowledge that I couldn't have children," she states flatly. "Never. Women are so afraid of that, but it's absolute nonsense.

"A man *senses* a sexy lady. He knows when she's looking, and it doesn't matter whether you've got that stuff inside or not. He can't see that it's not there. He's got the feeling already, and what's *important* is there, all right. That feeling, that aroused sexual feeling, is *there*. You could tell him you're Rin-Tin-Tin at that point, he doesn't really care. And it's nonsense for anybody to say that he does."

Of course, there are some men to whom children are very important, but at the age at which the vast majority of hysterectomy patients have to have their operations, most of those men have already fathered their broods.

A posthysterectomy patient is just not very likely to run across many men of her own age to whom new babies mean anything important at all. Sylvia didn't, nor did Diane (Chapter Eight), who decided to keep the information to herself unless she became seriously interested in a man who was caught up in the idea of beginning a family in his late forties. She didn't expect that she would.

After a few years, Sylvia met a man close to her own age with whom she is now very happy. The two of them make up one of those modern couples to whom children are somebody else's concern. "All of this business worked *for* me, not against me," Sylvia points out. "Think of the total freedom we have that other people don't have—the freedom of not having children, frankly. Wow, what a freedom that is!"

Finally, thirteen years after her hysterectomy, Sylvia came to the end of her gynecological problems when the last of her remaining ovary was removed because of a chocolate cyst (see Chapter Three). By that time, she was glad to be done with it. "The operation per se was a bore to me," she says. "By that time I had had seven of them, including the early D and C's. What a relief it was to know that there was nothing left for them to take out!"

This time, of course, she did have some physical reactions, primarily because, at forty-four, she was still too young for the natural menopause, and her internal hormone supply had stopped abruptly because of the surgery. Shortly after the operation, she began estrogen replacement therapy. But before the hormones came the gas.

Intestinal gas is a natural reaction of the body to any abdominal surgery, and gynecological patients seem to have more of it than others. For a few days immediately after the operation, while she was still in the hospital, Sylvia and her three roommates made a project—and, fortunately, a laughing matter—out of one more thing that could have brought on the blues if they had allowed it to.

"By that point, right after the operation," she relates, "nobody really gives a hoot any more about what has been cut out. The main, the one, and the only true thought in our minds at that point was to *get rid of that gas*. It's the most excruciating feeling—but it's laughable because you know what it is. You're not frightened by it, so you can turn your mind away from all those other bad thoughts and concentrate on this one goal. It's like a toothache that makes you forget your foot's sore—a counterirritant.

"It's a transference, of course, but a good one. You're not thinking about the sad side of life because your mind is totally engrossed in just one thing: the biggest possible *wind* in the world!

"Of course, it becomes hilarious because everybody's shyness of this problem is totally broken down. There we were, a quartet of lovely limousines, all creating this terrific air-pollution problem with our exhaust. When you hear one, you cheer and say, 'Did you do that? Boy, are you lucky!' And everyone laughs until their stitches hurt.

"It's amazing what the body does for you—now you're laughing and it's a joyous thing. Just by the act of doing that socially taboo thing—you know you're not supposed to go around 'doing that'—you're doing all the right things for your condition. You know the longer you just lie there, the worse it's going to get. So you get up and walk around, one of the best things you can do for yourself physically.

"We'd walk up and down the hall and check on each other and make reports: 'Boy, did I have a good one this morning!' It sounds like something out of the Body English

Manual—a bunch of women, all bent over, cracking up about their silly gas!"

After the gas was gone and she returned to the outside world, Sylvia went back to work very quickly, mainly because she didn't go along with the idea of lying around, getting bored, and continuing to feel like a patient. Now that her second ovary was gone, however, she did notice some disconcerting physical changes.

"After the last operation, I couldn't understand the tiredness, the overheating at night, the occasional insomnia. It's not like the old phrase 'hot flashes'—it's an overheating of the whole body and just . . . uncomfortable." Finally she mentioned her discomfort to her doctor, who promptly began her estrogen replacement therapy.

Sylvia takes a natural estrogen in pill form, one of the most popular with posthysterectomy patients. Fortunately, it seems to suit her perfectly. She takes one pill a day, every day for three weeks, then no pills at all for another week before resuming the cycle. She has had no side effects except for a slight bloating during her "off" week, a feeling she describes as "what used to be my before-period feeling." Once she started taking the pills, the overheating and nervous spells stopped and, she claims, "I felt like a new person within a week."

She did not gain weight and has no reason to expect to. As for sexual responsiveness, she reports happily that, "All those taboos are ridiculous—I feel just as sexy as I ever have."

Now, looking back over more than thirty years of gynecological problems and their solutions, Sylvia believes that it was all part of a natural progression toward a satisfying result. "I don't think whatever success and recognition I have achieved could ever have happened without all those experiences," she says reflectively. "Nature has a way of balancing itself out—you lose one thing, you gain something else.

"My philosophy, I guess, is just that things do work out for the best. I hate how corny that sounds, but it's true. All of this really has strengthened me. Of course, if I had read that in a book when I was sixteen, I would have thrown up at how maudlin it seems to be. But it does get you through all those battles, and you come out much stronger, much more aware of your own body and your own self, much more complete with yourself, even though you may have lost a little something inside that you've never even seen.

"You're forced to face life in a different way. And I think it's great what you receive in exchange for this giving up of little pieces of you.

"It makes you more tolerant, much more tolerant of other people. It also makes you smile at yourself when you start complaining about things—you stop and say to yourself, 'Hey, there, how easily we forget. What do you think you're doing with all this whining?' And things become very easy to do.

"Except for that one period, before the therapy made me see what was happening, I just haven't had the time to sit around and brood about things. You either deal with it well, or you fall apart, and falling apart was just a *bore*, frankly, and expensive. So you have to get out of it. You have to reach."

As Maude's husband said to her, after she had unburdened herself and he had succeeded in making her laugh, "Hey, Maude, look what just happened: You forgot to feel sorry for yourself. . . ."